Human Resources and Organizational Behavior

Cases in Health Services Management

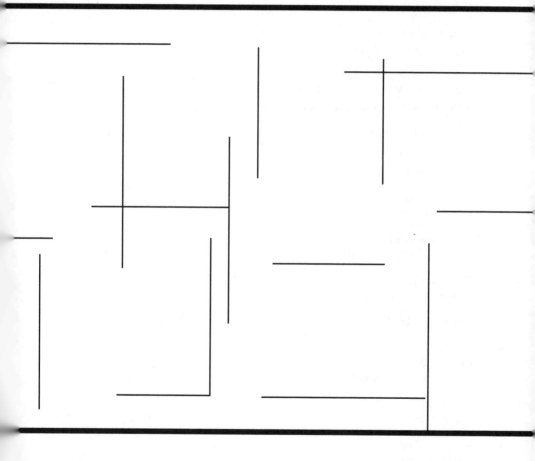

Human Resources and Organizational Behavior
Cases in Health Services Management

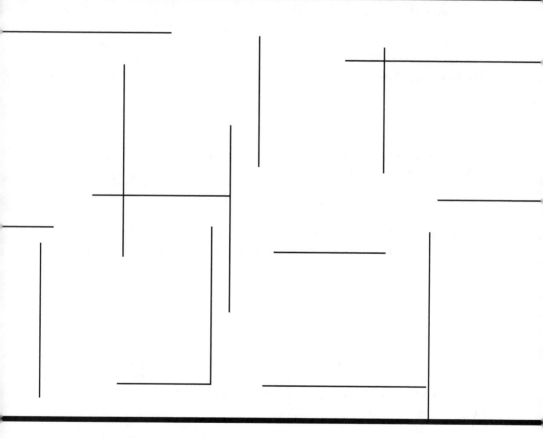

Anne Osborne Kilpatrick   James A. Johnson
With the assistance of Ann Hagins and Glenda Lee Thompson

Health Administration Press
Chicago, Illinois

03   02   5   4   3   2

Library of Congress Cataloging-in-Publication Data
Kilpatrick, Anne Osborne, 1945–
Human resources and organizational behavior: cases in health services
   management / by Anne Osborne Kilpatrick and James Allen Johnson.
      p.   cm.
   ISBN 1-56793-104-9 (alk. paper)
   1. Health facilities—Personnel management—Case studies.   2. Health
   services administration—Case studies   I. Johnson, James A., 1954–   .
   II. Title.
RA971.35.K54   1999
362.1'068'3—dc21   98-56539
                                                                        CIP

The paper used in this publication meets the minimum requirements of American National Standard for Information Sciences—Permanence of Paper for Printed Library Materials, ANSI Z39.48–1984.   ∞™

Health Administration Press
A division of the Foundation
   of the American College of
   Healthcare Executives
One North Franklin Street
Chicago, IL 60606-3491
(312) 424-2800

Association of University Programs
   in Health Administration
1110 Vermont Avenue, NW
Suite 220
Washington, D.C. 20005-3500
(202) 822-8550

CONTENTS

PREFACE

THE RAPID changes occurring in healthcare delivery and in organizations require healthcare professionals to respond in innovative ways to the competing demands and pressures from inside and outside their organization. The most pressing external and internal pressures include the following:

1. Increasing competition and the resulting need for dramatic improvements in organizational effectiveness. Managing financial, physical, and human resources efficiently and effectively is more than just a challenge; it is essential for organizational survival and growth. However, rapid growth and change have fostered attention to positive and negative growth management, and downsizing or resizing have become regular management tools. Finding the best way to change organizational structures and processes to enhance efficiency and effectiveness is a high priority in virtually all healthcare organizations. The implementation of such changes has important consequences for the morale and attitudes of healthcare workers as well as for organizational effectiveness as a whole.

2. Increasing complexity and size of organizations. Healthcare organizations are larger today and often more diversified. There has been a rapid growth of vertically integrated delivery systems, multi-institutional systems, large group practices, and healthcare holding companies. Many other kinds of alliances have also emerged, including collaborations among organizations that are considered competitors. Developing the organizational designs and the processes that will create the desired outcomes is a formidable challenge. In addition, the resulting complexity and overbureaucratization serve to isolate employees from both the organization and the competitive environment in which the institution must operate.

3. Rapid growth and the development of new market areas for healthcare. Growth and development of new market areas result in the need for innovative organizational and work-group designs to take advantage of the new opportunities and ongoing improvement and expansion of skills and knowledge for the healthcare professional. An increasing amount of specialization is required to provide a wide range of new services in market areas previously untapped by healthcare organizations.

4. Government involvement in controlling costs and regulating the healthcare industry. Reimbursement systems such as diagnosis-related groups have a direct effect on staffing and other human resource areas. Government funding of professional education and the regulation of health providers, including alternative providers, provide numerous challenges to the healthcare system.

5. Increasing professionalization of the workforce. Most of the allied health occupations are becoming professions with licensing or certification requirements, increased educational preparation requirements, codes of practice, and professional associations. The newly emerging professions are also being given more responsibility and greater decision-making authority. This change provides a challenge to the domains once dominated by physicians and administrators and calls for innovations in service delivery and decision-making processes.

6. Changing values of the workforce, particularly relative to lifestyle. Employees want to structure their own time as much as possible. Commitments outside of the workplace may receive higher priority than they once did. The dual career couple is rapidly becoming a social norm, and people have become much more mobile. Values within the workplace have changed as well; there is a greater expectation of rewards, autonomy, and the opportunity to influence the organization. Therefore, a growing number of healthcare institutions are reexamining the extent of their employee's involvement and influence. Some have developed new mechanisms that show promise for creating a more responsive organizational culture.

7. More concern with career development. Healthcare organizations are reexamining traditional assumptions about career paths and many are now providing alternative career opportunities, career counseling services, and career paths that are responsive to the particular needs of their employees. Much of the progress in this area has occurred in the field of nursing, where the desire to remain in the clinical path rather than managerial is fairly widespread.

8. Diversity in the workplace. As demographic changes affect the composition of the workforce, conflicts of culture, language, gender, and work patterns will increase. Discrimination and harassment have emerged as important issues for healthcare managers.

Numerous other pressures and social forces are placing demands on healthcare managers, including a shortage of certain health professionals, problems of pay equity, AIDS in the workplace, maldistribution of human resources (particularly physicians), deteriorating physical plants for many hospitals, and an aging population. What has become obvious in observing the changing environment of healthcare is that these changes and their subsequent demands have created the need for more institutional and managerial attention to organizational behavior and human resource planning, management, and development. Healthcare organizations must begin to take a long-term perspective in managing people, and more important, must acknowledge that human resources are an organization's most valued asset.

More than ten years ago, Joseph Califano signaled this need in the opening statement to his book *America's Health Care Revolution*: "A revolution in the American way of health is under way, and it's likely to be as far-reaching as any economic and social upheaval we have known." That statement has proven prophetic; the revolution has begun but is far from over. Part of the revolution involves changes in the way we work, changes in information and knowledge, changes in organizational structure and alignments, changes in professional authority, and changes in consumer demands. All of these present new problems and challenges for managers and behavioral scientists seeking to understand, influence, and manage healthcare organizations and employees in this new environment.

Purpose and Structure

This casebook is designed to help current and future healthcare professionals grapple with the challenges arising from the rapidly changing healthcare system. The cases are short enough to be easily integrated into a lecture format to give students practice with a specific topic; they are complex enough to allow rich discussions and varied interpretations. They can also be useful for professional development among working managers. (More information about pedagogic uses of cases is in the next section.)

The cases in this book are all related to key topics in healthcare human resources management and organizational behavior. Figures P.1 and P.2 will help instructors determine the specific topics relevant to each case. Figure P.1 categorizes the cases according to major topics in organizational behavior. (The topics are derived from the chapter titles of *Essentials of Health Care Management* by Stephen M. Shortell and Arnold D. Kaluzny.) Figure P.2 categorizes the cases according to major topics in healthcare human resources management. (The topics are derived from the chapter titles of the forthcoming *Managing Healthcare Human Resources* by James A. Johnson and Bruce J. Fried.) These matrices should help guide instructors in integrating these cases into their courses.

Using the Case Approach

The case approach to management and administration has been a valuable learning tool in schools of business and administration for decades. The case approach has several advantages:

- The cases simulate real-life situations.
- Actual problems that occur in healthcare or human services organizations are presented.
- Students are afforded the opportunity to practice decision making and problem analysis in a safe setting.
- The opportunity to present actual applications of theory to practice is afforded.

Students may identify various alternatives for solutions and are encouraged to look for as many options as possible. Additionally, they can analyze the probable outcomes of any decision made.

Students may use groups to discuss and solve the cases. This method is advantageous because it allows individual members to learn to work with others and to compare different responses to the same situations.

This book can also be used as a basis for role-playing. The safe environment of the classroom allows students to practice dealing with real-world problems and should help to equip them for actual situations in the future.

Instructors may also want students to write their analyses of cases as a way of helping students create systematic approaches to addressing management challenges. The outline in Table P.1 may be useful for case analyses. The outline suggests ways to diagnose the cases and to present the information, and includes criteria for evaluating the analyses.

Figure P.1   Relationship Between Cases and Organizational Behavior Text*

	Ch. 1 Organizational Theory and Health Services Management	Ch. 2 The Managerial Role	Ch. 3 Motivating People	Ch. 4 Leadership	Ch. 5 Conflict Management and Negotiation	Ch. 6 Managing Groups and Teams	Ch. 7 Work Design	Ch. 8 Coordination and Communication	Ch. 9 Power and Politics	Ch. 10 Organization Design	Ch. 11 Managing Strategic Alliances	Ch. 12 Organizational Innovation and Change	Ch. 13 Organizational Performance	Ch. 14 Strategy Making in Healthcare Organizations	Ch. 15 Creating and Managing the Future
Case 1: Death with Dignity								●							
Case 2: Sexual Harassment at St. Catherine	○			○	○				●						
Case 3: Managing the Maintenance Man	○			○				○							
Case 4: A Supervisor's Dilemma			○												
Case 5: Personal Feelings Versus Work Performance	○		○	○			●	●							●
Case 6: Inflated Statistics					●										
Case 7: A Subtle Case of Sexual Attraction					○										
Case 8: Paperwork Fiasco	●														
Case 9: Recurring Mistake	○					●									
Case 10: Who Will Work the Weekend?	○		○	●		●									
Case 11: We, the Counselors								●		○					
Case 12: The Independent Contractor								●							
Case 13: A Change of Leaders				○											
Case 14: Ugly Competition				○		·	○								
Case 15: Hostile Workplace			○		●	○									
Case 16: Same Hospital, Different Arrangement					○	●									
Case 17: A Case of Questionable Management					○										
Case 18: Impossible to Please															
Case 19: Combating Complacency															
Case 20: The Nursing Shortage															
Case 21: The Interim Director															
Case 22: Unprofessional Administration	○	○													
Case 23: The Overbearing Manager					●										
Case 24: Promoting Affirmatively	○	○	○												
Case 25: The Unexpected Problems											●		○		
Case 26: It's My Job!			○												
Case 27: The Evening-Shift Dilemma		○	●	○											
Case 28: The Abusive Patient		○		○	○										
Case 29: The Ostrich Employee						●									
Case 30: Harassment?					○										
Case 31: The Suspicious Performance Appraisals	○													●	
Case 32: Apathy . . . or Sabotage?												○	○	○	

Figure P.1 Relationship Between Cases and Organizational Behavior Text

	Ch. 1 Organizational Theory and Health Services Management	Ch. 2 The Managerial Role	Ch. 3 Motivating People	Ch. 4 Leadership	Ch. 5 Conflict Management and Negotiation	Ch. 6 Managing Groups and Teams	Ch. 7 Work Design	Ch. 8 Coordination and Communication	Ch. 9 Power and Politics	Ch. 10 Organization Design	Ch. 11 Managing Strategic Alliances	Ch. 12 Organizational Innovation and Change	Ch. 13 Organizational Performance	Ch. 14 Strategy Making in Healthcare Organizations	Ch. 15 Creating and Managing the Future
Case 33: Broken Promises		○	●												
Case 34: How Do You End an Unprofitable Business Relationship?											○	●		○	○
Case 35: Is this a Case of Discrimination?		○	○	○				●							○
Case 36: The Problem with the Temporary Pool		○							●	●					
Case 37: The Revolving Door		●	○	○									○		
Case 38: The Obstinate Senior Technician															
Case 39: Insubordination	●	○	●						●						
Case 40: The Substandard Employee			○			●									
Case 41: The Consolidation of Laboratories								○							
Case 42: The New Computer System								○				○	○	○	
Case 43: Problems in the Nursing Department		○			○	●		○		●					
Case 44: Must I Treat an AIDS Patient?		○											○		
Case 45: Conflict Between Managers					●	○									
Case 46: The Delegator								○				●		●	●
Case 47: When the Appointed Disappoints	○	○													
Case 48: Simplifying an Organizational Chart		○													
Case 49: The First Meeting												●		●	●
Case 50: The Blood Bank Dilemma	○	○		○											
Case 51: Uncooperative Chiefs									○						
Case 52: A Good Relationship Turned Sour									○				○		
Case 53: Waiting for Retirement					●										
Case 54: Retaining Technicians	●														
Case 55: Employee of the Year							●								
Case 56: Who's the Boss?					○					●					
Case 57: Insult to Injury?															
Case 58: Disciplining the Abusive Charge Nurse															
Case 59: The Flirtatious Physician		○													
Case 60: The Counterproductive Employee	○														
Case 61: A Quality Improvement Program Intervention	○	○											○		

Legend: ○ = directly related ● = indirectly related
*Shortell, S. M., and A. D. Kaluzney. 1997. *Essentials of Health Care Management*. Albany, NY: Delmar Publications.

Figure P.2 Relationship Between Cases and Human Resources Text*

	Ch. 1 Strategic Management of Human Resources	Ch. 2 The Health Professions	Ch. 3 The Healthcare Manpower Labor Market	Ch. 4 The Legal Environment of H.R. Management	Ch. 5 Job Design and Job Analysis	Ch. 6 Human Resources Planning in Organizations	Ch. 7 Recruitment, Selection, and Socialization	Ch. 8 Employee Separations	Ch. 9 Performance Management	Ch. 10 Human Resources Development and Training	Ch. 11 Compensation and Incentives	Ch. 12 Employee Benefits	Ch. 13 Health and Safety in the Workplace	Ch. 14 Employee and Management Rights	Ch. 15 Employee Relations and Communications	Ch. 16 Working with Organized Labor	Ch. 17 Information and Evaluation of the H.R. Function
Case 1: Death with Dignity																	
Case 2: Sexual Harassment at St. Catherine				○										○	○		
Case 3: Managing the Maintenance Man														●	○		
Case 4: A Supervisor's Dilemma									○								
Case 5: Personal Feelings Versus Work Performance					●	○								○			
Case 6: Inflated Statistics																	
Case 7: A Subtle Case of Sexual Attraction														○			
Case 8: Paperwork Fiasco															○		
Case 9: Recurring Mistake														●	○		
Case 10: Who Will Work the Weekend?														○	○		
Case 11: We, the Counselors				●	●												
Case 12: The Independent Contractor																	
Case 13: A Change of Leaders		○				○			○								
Case 14: Ugly Competition		○															
Case 15: Hostile Workplace									○					●			
Case 16: Same Hospital, Different Arrangement																	
Case 17: A Case of Questionable Management																	
Case 18: Impossible to Please															○		
Case 19: Combating Complacency																	
Case 20: The Nursing Shortage																	
Case 21: The Interim Director																	
Case 22: Unprofessional Administration		○															
Case 23: The Overbearing Manager																	
Case 24: Promoting Affirmatively		○												○	○		
Case 25: The Unexpected Problems		○				○								○			
Case 26: It's My Job!					●												
Case 27: The Evening-Shift Dilemma							●							●			
Case 28: The Abusive Patient								○					●	○			
Case 29: The Ostrich Employee					●												
Case 30: Harassment?				○													
Case 31: The Suspicious Performance Appraisals				○	○				○								
Case 32: Apathy . . . or Sabotage?									○								

Figure P.2 Relationship Between Cases and Human Resources Text

	Ch. 1 Strategic Management of Human Resources	Ch. 2 The Health Professions	Ch. 3 The Healthcare Manpower Labor Market	Ch. 4 The Legal Environment of H.R. Management	Ch. 5 Job Design and Job Analysis	Ch. 6 Human Resources Planning in Organizations	Ch. 7 Recruitment, Selection, and Socialization	Ch. 8 Employee Separations	Ch. 9 Performance Management	Ch. 10 Human Resources Development and Training	Ch. 11 Compensation and Incentives	Ch. 12 Employee Benefits	Ch. 13 Health and Safety in the Workplace	Ch. 14 Employee and Management Rights	Ch. 15 Employee Relations and Communications	Ch. 16 Working with Organized Labor	Ch. 17 Information and Evaluation of the H.R. Function
Case 33: Broken Promises	O																
Case 34: How Do You End an Unprofitable Business Relationship?	O		●						O								
Case 35: Is This a Case of Discrimination?															O		
Case 36: The Problem with the Temporary Pool	O		O														
Case 37: The Revolving Door	●					O									O		
Case 38: The Obstinate Senior Technician																	
Case 39: Insubordination						●	O		O								
Case 40: The Substandard Employee									O			O					
Case 41: The Consolidation of Laboratories						O										●	
Case 42: The New Computer System	O								●								
Case 43: Problems in the Nursing Department															O		
Case 44: Must I Treat an AIDS Patient?													O				
Case 45: Conflict Between Managers															O		
Case 46: The Delegator																	
Case 47: When the Appointed Disappoints									O								O
Case 48: Simplifying an Organizational Chart						O											O
Case 49: The First Meeting																	●
Case 50: The Blood Bank Dilemma																	O
Case 51: Uncooperative Chiefs																	
Case 52: A Good Relationship Turned Sour																	O
Case 53: Waiting for Retirement																O	
Case 54: Retaining Technicians	O	●			●												O
Case 55: Employee of the Year																	
Case 56: Who's the Boss?																●	●
Case 57: Insult to Injury?															O		
Case 58: Disciplining the Abusive Charge Nurse														O			
Case 59: The Flirtatious Physician																●	
Case 60: The Counterproductive Employee														O	●		
Case 61: A Quality Improvement Program Intervention									O								

Legend: O = directly related   ● = indirectly related
*Johnson, J. A., and B. Fried. 1999. *Managing Healthcare Human Resources*. Chicago: Health Administration Press.

Table P.1   Sample Outline for Written Case Analysis

I. Major Facts

Facts may be reported in narrative form or may be outlined. These should include the most important and pertinent incidents in the situation. (Do not simply restate the entire case.)

II. Problem(s)

The facts of the case reveal one or more problems that require attention. Indicate those problems and briefly explain their importance. A good place to look for problems is to begin with structural questions: Has an organizational chart been provided? If not, create one. What are the reporting relationships? Does the affected employee report to more than one person? Are written policies or procedures described? Is a legal issue involved, or is it primarily a problem of communication, conflict, roles, or other less tangible issues?

III. Alternative Solutions and Probable Outcomes

A principle, "every action will have a reaction," pertains here. Analyze optional courses of action and the probable outcomes of each. This is one of the most important parts of the analysis. Remember that a decision not to act or to do nothing is always an alternative. However, doing nothing also has repercussions—sometimes worse repercussions than any other action. Identify as many alternatives as possible, even if some appear farfetched.

IV. Recommended Solution and Probable Outcome

This section should include the recommended action, justification for the action, how that action would be implemented, and the probable outcome(s). While some of this information has been included in previous sections, it is still important to present the recommendation in its final form and to justify its selection.

Evaluation Criteria

Criteria for evaluation might include the following:

- Organization: Did students answer all the parts of the assignment in a logical sequence?
- Integration: Did students incorporate readings, including theories, research, and models, into the analysis?
- Management practice: Did students consider several alternatives? What methods did they present to assess the effectiveness of their decision(s)?
- Composition: Is the writing technically correct and stylistically appropriate?

Acknowledgments

The editors would like to thank the following for their valuable contributions to this book: Penny Adsit; Lindsey Davis Alley; Maria K. Anderson; Jan Booth; Jerry K. Burik; Stacy Anthony Byrd; Reginald D.

Evans; Pamela Fleming; Mark K. Floro; Joseph G. France, Jr.; April P. Garrett; J. Daniel Gentry; Lisa Grubb; Jamie Guin; Sara Ann Hagins; Suzanne Hogsett; Anita H. Hughes; Diane Hunter; Donna Hurley-Howell; Gerard C. Jebaily; Harriet Jeffords; Sharon Faulconer Kieffer; Yana Kistler; Moha Laag; Ann S. Lambert; Stephen T. Lesieur; Eileen M. Loewenthal; Gary Scot Mitchell; Stacy T. Mullins; Wendy R. Munn; William A. Munn; Nancy D. Pope; Wanda Prevatte; Mary Jo Repasky; Keith Rodgers; Ellen Romani; Ruth E. Ross; Susan Sams; John M. Sanders; Judy Shelton; Andrea Shirey; Patty C. Slay; Mark Spencer; Carol A. Tesh; Penny Winn Tisdale; and Eugene Toomer, Jr.

References

Califano, J. A. 1986. *America's Health Care Revolution: Who Lives, Who Dies, Who Pays.* New York: Random House.

Johnson, J.A., and B. Fried. *Managing Healthcare Human Resources.* Chicago: Health Administration Press (in press).

Shortell, S.M., and A.D. Kaluzny. 1997. *Essentials of Health Care Management.* Albany, NY: Delmar Publishers.

1

Death with Dignity

D R. BELLAMY, the medical director of Mercy Hospital in South Carolina, has asked you, the hospital's social worker, to call an emergency meeting of the hospital's ethics committee to address a difficult situation that occurred over the past weekend. Dr. Bellamy was notified of the situation by Donna, a respiratory therapist, who was very upset and demanded that the problem be resolved. Donna is angry because she believes that Mercy Hospital does not provide its attending and resident physicians with adequate information about the South Carolina Death with Dignity Act, which became law in 1986, and that this lack of information served to exacerbate an already difficult situation.

Before you call the members of the ethics committee, you decide to speak to Donna to hear her version of the story. Donna explains to you that an emergency page went out at 5 p.m. Saturday to the code team, of which she was a member that day, for Mrs. Brownlee, a 78-year-old patient on the oncology floor who had suffered a respiratory arrest and a cardiac insult. Donna tells you that when she arrived at the scene, resuscitation efforts were underway, and the patient's daughter was pleading with the physicians to stop. Several hospital employees, including nurses, doctors, and ancillary staff, heard the woman say, "That's my mother in there, and I don't want her on a respirator. *Please*, don't put her on a respirator!"

Donna goes on to explain that the doctors who were performing the resuscitation ignored the daughter's request, closed the door in her face, and sent a junior resident out to speak to her. Donna heard the resident say to the patient's daughter, "Ma'am, I'm sorry that we have to do this, but if we don't, we might get sued."

The daughter replied, "But that's my mother. She's 78 years old and is suffering from terminal cancer. I don't want her on a respirator."

The resident answered, "I'm sorry, but we have to do it to cover ourselves."

The patient was taken to the only open intensive care unit bed and placed on full life-support services.

Earlier, when you spoke to Dr. Bellamy, she informed you that the patient's family will attend the meeting of the ethics committee and will request that Mrs. Brownlee be removed from all life-support equipment despite opposition from her attending physician, an oncologist.

Dr. Bellamy mentioned that the patient had a living will on her chart and requested that you determine whether this puts Mercy Hospital in liability. She also asks you to consider whether the hospital should offer to cover the part of the patient's costs that is not covered by her insurance.

Discussion Questions

1. What are the ethical considerations of the case?
2. What are the legal implications of the case?
3. As the hospital social worker, what actions would you recommend to Dr. Bellamy?
4. Would your recommendation be different if you were the medical director?

Sexual Harassment at St. Catherine

F ATIMA WAS hired as a registered nurse in the maternity department of St. Catherine Hospital on July 1, immediately after her graduation from nursing school. Her husband, Ali, had been working as a lab technician at St. Catherine for more than five years. Fatima was happy with her job and enjoyed socializing with her coworkers. Her only complaint was that she was assigned to the night shift while her husband worked the day shift.

After Fatima had been working at St. Catherine for three months, Ali asked his boss to speak to the hospital director about the possibility of getting Fatima reassigned to the day shift. He did, and two days later Fatima's shift was changed. When Omar, the nursing supervisor, heard about the change in Fatima's work schedule, he was angry that he had not been included in the decision-making process. He also began to pay attention to Fatima for the first time since she began working at St. Catherine.

Omar began making unusually frequent visits to the maternity department, especially the area where Fatima worked. The head nurse in the maternity department, Anne, noticed the frequent visits but didn't speculate about the reason for them.

On October 20, Omar called Fatima into his office. They had the following conversation:

Omar: I asked you to come here so I could find out more about you before assigning you more responsibility.
Fatima: More responsibility? What do you mean?

Omar: Well, I was thinking of promoting you to head nurse of the maternity department.

Fatima: Head nurse? Anne is more qualified for that position than I am; she has far more experience. Besides, I need to work here for at least one year before I'm eligible for a promotion.

Omar: I know the rules. But, you see, I have a lot of influence at the hospital. I can persuade the director very easily. Besides, Anne has a record of being hostile toward hospital administration.

Fatima: Thank you for the offer, but I don't think I'm qualified for the position. I need to get back to my work now, if we're finished here.

Omar: OK, but give my offer some more thought. This is a great opportunity for you, and I don't want you to miss it because I care for you. Oh, one more thing, could you please keep this conversation confidential?

After this conversation, Omar's visits to the maternity department became even more frequent. On November 15, Omar came to the department at 6 p.m., after most of the nurses had gone home. Fatima was still there, getting ready to leave. This conversation followed:

Omar: I'm glad you're alone. I just want to ask if you have some free time next week. I'd like us to spend some time together . . .

Fatima: Stop it! You are my supervisor, and you are supposed to set an example of honesty and respect. Besides, we're both married. Please excuse me; my husband is waiting for me.

Fatima left feeling upset and embarrassed. Because of her religious and social beliefs, however, she chose not to tell anybody about what happened, even her husband. The following day, still upset, she called in sick. Omar, angry, immediately reported her absence to the director.

One week later, Fatima was transferred to the intensive care unit and a written warning was placed in her permanent record. Fatima, with only a few months of nursing experience, was not prepared for the complexity of the work in her new position. The head nurse of the intensive care unit, Renee, was instructed by Omar to notify him in writing of every instance in which Fatima was not able to perform her new duties. Omar provided the discipline committee with copies of these documents and used them to convince the members of the committee that Fatima had failed to carry out her assignments properly. As a result, Fatima was transferred to a small rural hospital located 95 miles from St. Catherine.

In July, at the end of her first year of employment, Fatima received a copy of her performance evaluation. It stated, "After a one-year probationary period, Fatima's performance did not meet the necessary requirements; therefore, we are recommending the prolongation of her probationary period for an additional year." The performance evaluation was signed by the director of St. Catherine, Omar, and Renee. Fatima refused to sign and decided to file official sexual harassment charges against Omar.

Discussion Questions

1. How could this situation have been handled differently?
2. Is Omar the only person at fault in this case? Do the head nurses and hospital director share in any of the responsibility?
3. If you were assigned responsibility to research this case, what kinds of questions would you ask the parties involved?

Managing the Maintenance Man

T HE RANDOLF Society is a privately owned organization that comprises several subsidiary corporations including a 40-bed hospital and a venture capital company. The venture capital company has a real estate division that manages two physician office buildings owned by the Randolf Society.

Jim is the on-site maintenance coordinator of the real estate division. His primary responsibility is the daily maintenance and management of the two physician office buildings. He was appointed to this position based on his favorable performance evaluation and his ten-year experience at the hospital's maintenance department. He works unsupervised but reports directly to his immediate supervisor Carol, a licensed property manager and corporate accountant for the venture capital company. Carol approves his work requisitions and supply purchases.

Cost-containment efforts by the company have recently resulted in the shifting of the cleaning and maintenance service contract of the physician office buildings to the hospital's environmental services department. This shift brought in Paula, the director of environmental services, with whom Jim has conflicts—conflicts that stem from his frequent absenteeism, insubordination, and confusion about who is now his manager and how to prioritize his duties. Jim expressed his discontent to the unaware Carol, who subsequently asked Paula about it; Carol determined that Paula's expectations of Jim were reasonable and justified.

However, of more concern to Carol is that Jim may be involved in some shady activities occurring in the physician offices. Because of Jim's frequent absenteeism, Carol was forced to assign a substitute, Tom, to respond to calls when Jim could not. During the days that Tom was on duty, he received several message pages from Jim's "friends" requesting money, and he noticed numerous suspicious-looking people by the back entrance who abruptly left the area when he approached. In addition, several physicians reported office break-ins and complained of missing prescription notepads. Jim holds the only master key to the offices. Carol thinks that Jim may have a drug problem.

As Jim's immediate supervisor, Carol must make an informed decision about whether to reprimand or to fire Jim based on these events. She cannot base her decision on suspicions and assumptions alone; she must rely on facts and then use the company's policy and protocols (for example, hospital policy mandates drug testing only for new employees) to guide her in making the best decision.

Discussion Questions

1. Are there problems with the organizational structure of the Randolf Society? Explain.
2. How should Jim's disinterest in his job—apparent in his frequent absenteeism and the possibility of a drug problem—be dealt with?
3. What steps should be taken to preserve the relationship between the real estate division and the physicians who occupy the office buildings if the burglary problems remain unsolved?

4

A Supervisor's Dilemma

MARY WAS hired as a night clerk at a hospital's laboratory. Her job duties included answering the phone, taking requests, and receiving and logging laboratory samples into the computer system for processing. Before she began her night shift, she received ample training during the day. Her supervisors considered this training to be sufficient for performing her night duties.

However, when Mary started the night shift, computer errors started to occur. These mistakes were attributed to Mary's lack of experience with the computer system; therefore, she was given additional training by her immediate and department supervisors during her regular shift. However, the added training did not help and Mary continued making more mistakes. Furthermore, Mary did not seem willing to remedy the situation; instead, she denied the mistakes, made excuses to get out of the laboratory even at extremely busy times, and frequently called in sick or took days off without checking the schedule. As a result, Mary's night-shift coworker was often left performing two jobs, and animosity among fed-up staff members increased.

Because Mary's immediate supervisor, Eunice, could not resolve Mary's issues, the department supervisor, Dorene, had to intervene. Dorene counseled Mary and advised her of the disciplinary actions that would follow. The hospital policy was first to counsel the employee; if the problem continued, the employee would be written up and the report would be placed in the employee's file. Termination would occur after three documented incidents. Mary denied any problems.

Despite Dorene's warnings and a counseling session with the entire night shift, Mary continued to create problems and Eunice continued to be incapable of resolving them. As a result, both Mary and Eunice were written up. As time went on, it became evident that Mary was completely disinterested in her job.

When a new position opened in a different area of the hospital, Mary asked for a transfer and was offered the position, which she promptly accepted. Mary's final performance evaluation at the laboratory documented all the problems that had occurred while she was in Dorene's department. Mary confronted Dorene and stated that the evaluation was all lies; she never admitted to making any mistakes and even said that she had been complimented by her coworkers on her high performance and ability to handle her job.

Now, Dorene is torn between giving an honest reference that will damage Mary's chance of getting the job and giving a good reference that will help Mary get the job, hasten her departure from the unit, and finally resolve the long-running conflict between them.

Discussion Questions

1. How should Mary, as a difficult employee, be handled?
2. How should Eunice, as the immediate supervisor, establish her authority?
3. What would you do if you were the supervisor faced with Dorene's dilemma?
4. What long-term effect would giving a good reference have for Dorene and the unit?

5

Personal Feelings Versus Work Performance

MARTHA, A department manager at Amesville Hospital, hired Jane as the department secretary. Martha and Jane were the only employees in the department at that time. When Jane was hired, Martha assured her that the department was growing and that, with her college education and experience, she had the potential for career advancement if she worked diligently.

Six months later, Leonard, a colleague from another department who had the same level of education but less experience, was transferred to Jane and Martha's department and given the same salary as Jane. Immediately, Martha showed signs of favoritism toward Leonard. Within the following three years, Leonard, despite poor performance appraisals, was promoted three times and was given major pay increases. Jane achieved superior performance evaluations and awards, but merely received cost-of-living salary increases. As time went on, four more employees were added to the department, which increased Jane's workload and responsibility; however, she was not promoted.

Jane approached Martha on several occasions about the apparent discrepancies in the promotion patterns at the department. Although Martha agreed that Leonard was barely meeting standards and acknowledged that Jane was doing most of his work, she also stated that promoting a male was "easier." In addition, Martha told Jane that recommending a change of job description that would incorporate Jane's management-level work would take time. Tired of doing Leonard's job and not getting credit, Jane was pirated away by another healthcare agency that offered her a management position and appropriate pay.

Unfortunately, the healthcare agency closed after a year and a half. Because Jane had a good reputation at Amesville Hospital and desired a more secure position, she sought employment there again. After hearing that Leonard was leaving his post at Amesville, Jane asked Martha how she would feel if she applied for Leonard's job when he left. Martha said she could not think of a more qualified person.

In the meantime, Jane accepted a job in the department as a low-grade clerk typist just to have an income. Martha seemed pleased to have Jane back and said her knowledge of the department made her perfect to take charge of a new computer project. Jane was given many management-level projects to work on, but her responsibilities were never clarified. Jane was torn over whether to perform as a clerk and show initiative or to perform as a manager and run the project, which would show Martha that Jane was capable. It was never clearly stated that any project was given to her to manage completely, and Martha even told Jane that one of the projects Jane had been given had been given to Martha by the hospital director with specific instructions not to delegate the project. Because Jane worked under the department secretary, she found it difficult to manage the projects without going over her boss or creating conflicts. When Jane asked Martha to clarify her position, Martha always either did not have time or acted as if Jane were incompetent for asking such questions. As time went by, Jane became increasingly frustrated with Martha's unprofessional attitude toward her.

When Leonard finally left his position, several applicants were interviewed, but none had Jane's qualifications. At Jane's interview, Martha asked her in an irritated voice, "What do you think you have done in the past three months to prove that you can handle Leonard's job?" At that moment, Jane felt that she had been set up to fail in those months and realized that Martha had never considered her for Leonard's position. Martha continued to criticize Jane about her weaknesses and enumerated all the projects and responsibilities that she had failed to accomplish. Trying to be professional, Jane told Martha that she should know her work habits well enough to realize that she would not knowingly neglect important details. When Jane asked why she was not told that she was expected to handle the projects in their entirety, Martha replied, "Well, I couldn't exactly *say* that."

Several days later, Martha told Jane that she was not strong enough for Leonard's position and another female hospital employee, who had no experience and a reputation for being a mediocre employee, was hired instead. Jane started applying for positions in other departments of the hospital but was warned by Martha that she had to complete the computer project before she left the department.

Discussion Questions

1. Was Jane treated unfairly?
2. What should Jane's course of action be?
3. What are the major problems in the department's management?

Inflated Statistics

C ATHERINE IS the personnel specialist at Vaughn Hospital. In the past year, she has been informed by six employees of questionable practices and unprofessional treatment of employees in the patient recreation service department, where the staff turnover rate is high.

Three employees stated that they had been instructed by the recreation coordinator, Matthew, to inflate statistics concerning the number of recreation and special activities and the number of participating volunteers and patients. According to staff, Matthew informed them that all hospitals inflated their statistics because the numbers ensured jobs in the department, but he failed to mention that these statistics also determined the hospital's budget and his salary.

In addition, orders for supplies and funding from special accounts were written up as if they were used for designated activities but were in fact being applied to other purposes. According to the secretary of the department, Matthew was using a VCR and a portable radio/tape recorder—one purchased for hospital use only—in his home.

All of these employees came to Catherine after they had resigned from their jobs in the department. Another staff member reported being threatened for refusing to apply for a vacant position within the department. Allegedly Matthew warned the employee that her current position might be abolished if she complained.

The employees indicated to Catherine that they wanted the allegations on record but were concerned about the repercussions of a formal grievance. They expressed concern that Matthew's prestige in the healthcare industry would affect their careers if they came forward.

Discussion Questions

1. Is Matthew involved in criminal activities?
2. Why are so many employees afraid of reporting obvious wrongdoing?
3. What should Catherine do?
4. What should the employees do?

7

A Subtle Case of Sexual Attraction

EVE IS the administrative resident at a for-profit hospital. She is energetic and hard working, has excellent communication skills, and fits well within the organization. During her first months, Eve worked very well with the administrative staff and was mentored by the president of operations.

Eve continued to thrive in her position and caught the attention of Monica, the vice president of operations, with whom Eve had been working closely. Monica became another mentor to Eve by helping her with projects, counseling her about careers, including her in upper-level management meetings, inviting her to social events and functions both in and out of the hospital, and asking her to come as a companion to out-of-town meetings that according to Monica would benefit Eve's future career. Monica also assured Eve that she could be instrumental in keeping Eve in an administrative position once the residency was completed.

Eve felt increasingly uncomfortable with Monica's attentions and started distancing herself by refusing the social invitations and business meetings. However, when Eve declined Monica's invitations, Monica began to pout and show resentment toward Eve. Monica also started criticizing Eve's job performance and appeared to exclude her from hospital staff meetings. Feeling unhappy and awkward about the conflict, Eve finally approaches you, the personnel director, for advice.

Discussion Questions

1. Is this a case of sexual harrassment or attraction? What is the difference?
2. As a personnel director, what advice would you give Eve? Monica?
3. How could this situation be avoided?

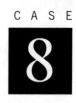
Paperwork Fiasco

C OUNTY GENERAL Memorial Hospital is a 75-bed rural hospital with a patient population of mostly elderly heart-attack victims. Because of its remote location, the hospital loses money every year and has difficulty retaining trained personnel.

The midnight shift at the hospital's laboratory consists of two people: Sally, a specimen processor, and Andy, an experienced medical technologist. Sally, who has little technical training, is responsible for receiving patient specimens, entering test requests on the computer, and forwarding the specimens to Andy. Andy performs the tests and enters the test results on the computer.

One Saturday night, Sally received a specimen with neither a label nor a test request card. Not wanting to fill out an incident report, she passed the specimen on to Andy. Andy reluctantly called the ward where the specimen originated and reminded the clerk, Patty, that it was against hospital policy for the lab to process unlabeled specimens with no request cards.

Patty told Andy she was "too busy" to label the specimen and that it needed to be tested immediately because of a medical emergency. Andy said that he would test it after proper paperwork was completed. Patty became angry and verbally abusive, and minutes later she stumbled into the laboratory with bloodshot eyes and smelling of alcohol. She demanded that the test be done right away, but Andy insisted that he still needed paperwork and threatened Patty that he would write an incident report. Shocked at the prospect of losing her job, Patty left the hospital. Andy did not conduct the test on the unlabeled specimen.

The patient to whom the specimen belonged died. The nursing supervisor, Cynthia, believed that if the test results had come back in a timely fashion, they might have saved the patient. Therefore Cynthia has written a formal report recommending that Andy be fired.

Discussion Questions

1. If you were the laboratory supervisor, what would you do about (1) Patty, the ward clerk; (2) Andy, the medical technologist; and (3) Sally, the specimen processor?
2. As lab supervisor, how will you respond to the nursing supervisor's report and recommendation?
3. What are the most significant human-relations issues in this case?
4. How would you improve organizational effectiveness after this incident?

Recurring Mistake

J OAN IS an 86-year-old woman who came to Colly County Memorial Hospital with dyspnea, fever, chills, and a persistent cough. She was diagnosed as having pneumonia, underlying conditions of malnutrition, and Alzheimer's disease, and she needed to be admitted into the hospital for medical management.

At the time of her arrival, the hospital was filled to capacity, but a bed would be available within an hour as a discharge was in process on the medical/surgical unit. Admitting orders were initiated in the emergency room, and Joan was taken to the radiology department for a chest x-ray while waiting for a room. The radiology department was busy and operating with less than full staff because three workers were out sick. It was two o'clock, and no staff had been able to eat lunch.

A registered technician, Pamela, wheeled Joan to one of the x-ray rooms, closed the door, and proceeded to lift Joan from her wheelchair and hoist her onto the examination table. Pamela knew that she was breaking the hospital policy requiring two technicians per patient. After the x-ray, Pamela assisted Joan from the examination table to the wheelchair, but during the transfer, Joan lost her balance and fell to the floor. Joan complained of a slight hip pain while Pamela was helping her up, but Pamela decided not to write an incident report in hopes that Joan would become confused about the fall. She then made arrangements for Joan to be taken to her room.

Two hours later, Joan's daughter notified the nurse that Joan had told her about the fall and the pain in her hip. The daughter demanded to know when the fall had occurred and why she had not been notified.

Joan underwent a hip examination that showed a fracture had resulted from the fall.

Pamela denied any knowledge of the incident. Further investigation into Pamela's background revealed that she had been terminated from her previous job because of a similar incident. However, Pamela had recorded a different reason on her job application at Colly County Memorial Hospital.

Discussion Questions

1. If you were Pamela's supervisor, which issues would you address?
2. What are the possible outcomes of this incident for (1) you as the supervisor, (2) Pamela, (3) the radiology department, and (4) the hospital?

Who Will Work the Weekend?

BRENDA IS the chemistry supervisor in a medium-sized community hospital. She supervises four technicians who rotate weekends on a two-on/two-off schedule. Two of her employees, Carol and Ellen, recently had an explosive fight about an upcoming weekend schedule—a fight that angered Carol so much that she threatened to resign.

The fight started when Ellen asked Carol to switch weekends so that Ellen could go on a trip to the Bahamas in two weeks. She had been invited by a friend and the dates were set. Ellen could not ask the other two technicians because one was already scheduled to work that weekend and the other had a previously planned engagement. Ellen knew Carol didn't have any previous appointments, so she did not think it was going to be a problem. Carol, on the other hand, took offense at Ellen's request and assumption about her weekend plans and claimed that she disapproved of switching schedules. (Carol had previously missed her brother's wedding so that she did not have to ask anyone to replace her.) Although Ellen was apologetic about the fight, she felt that she deserved the time off because she had never asked for vacation time in her two years at the job. Carol had never asked anyone to cover for her, so she did not think she owed anyone favors.

Brenda's policy about switching schedules is that her staff members are responsible for finding their own replacements and then informing her of changes. Brenda does not work on weekends at the request of her supervisor, and she does not fill in because she does not want her staff to expect it. Now she needs to find a replacement for the weekend and, most important, resolve the conflict between Carol and Ellen.

Discussion Questions

1. If you were Brenda, what would you do?
2. Should the weekend policy be changed to better suit the needs of the staff? How?

We, the Counselors

AMHERST PSYCHIATRIC Institute's nursing staff is composed of nurses and mental health counselors who provide 24-hour direct inpatient care. All nurses at Amherst have a state license and one of three educational accomplishments: a two-year hospital diploma, a two-year associate degree in nursing, or a four-year bachelor's degree in nursing. All mental health counselors are required to have a four-year bachelor's degree, preferably in the social science field, and some hold master's degrees in counseling or psychology.

The job responsibilities of the nurses and counselors are quite similar. In addition to their primary role of establishing a therapeutic relationship with patients, mental health counselors, like nurses, are required to take vital signs, give bed baths, assist with patients' activities of daily living (ADLs), and administer catheters as needed. Because the psychiatric patient usually requires less invasive therapy and supportive care than do medical/surgical patients, few distinctions are noticed in the routine function of the staff.

Working relationships between the nurses and counselors appear harmonious most of the time; minor conflicts over job duties are quickly and quietly settled by the unit nurse manager.

For the past year, the attrition rate among the counselors has been increasing steadily, but neither the unit nurse manager nor the director of nursing for the department have questioned the staff about the possible reasons for the turnover. Vacancies are usually filled immediately to adjust the patient-to-staff ratio.

The unit nurse manager informs the mental health counselor applicants that (1) the position does not offer an opportunity for career advancement within the department; (2) a working unity exists between the nurses and counselors to coordinate and deliver quality care; and (3) staff members are encouraged to resolve their own conflicts before approaching management.

Unknown to staff members and the nursing administration, the mental health counselors have formed a separate action group outside the work environment to discuss their dissatisfaction concerning their roles and responsibilities and the conflicts that exist with the staff nurses as well as their common feelings of perceived lack of value by nurses and administration. The counselors have agreed to present the problems affecting their morale and job performance to the nursing staff and administration and have chosen a spokesperson to voice their concerns at a meeting of counselors, nurses, and administration. The presentation follows.

We, the mental health counselors, are confused about our role within the nursing department. We perceive that we are made to feel subordinate to nurses in patient care areas such as counseling, even though many of us have a wealth of knowledge and experience in this area of patient care. We feel our efforts are undervalued and often go unrecognized by the nursing administration.

We do not want to take anything away from the nurses; rather, we would like to share equally in those areas of patient care in which we are qualified. It appears as if the administration continually seeks ways to expand and empower the role of nurses while excluding counselors from consideration for duties that may require more authority. Indeed our responsibilities at times have been further diminished. For many years, mental health counselors were responsible for processing patient admission and discharge procedures except for gathering intake physical information and examinations. Suddenly, we were given notice not to administer these responsibilities because of JCAHO's requirement that an RN must perform and document these duties. Yet our requests for documentation to support this change went unanswered, and now, six months later, we have been allowed to resume these duties without an explanation.

We are led to believe that nurses, like mental health counselors, share similar duties for the caring of patients. We also recognize that some techniques and interventions are specific for nurses; however, when daily assignments are made for patient care, mental health counselors inevitably are assigned to bedridden patients who require primary nursing care. We expected a sharing of duties.

continued

During our staff retreat, an announcement was made to staff nurses and mental health counselors about a possible pay increase of 50 cents an hour to occur soon. Later, we learned that only nurses were granted this raise. Again, no consideration was given to counselors as valued members of the nursing department.

Memos addressed to "All Nursing Staff" are passed individually to nurses. Counselors are left to learn of department policy changes through staff nurses.

Participation in team meetings is another area in which we feel we are unfairly excluded. Although these meetings are said to be open to counselors, in reality we are left to staff the unit while nurses attend the meetings. How are we to be team members when we share unequally in the team process?

As one mental health counselor expressed, "I don't think the nurses respect and trust our decision making. In a way their actions indicate we are not qualified. In fact, on matters of assessing a patient's mental health, I am equally if not more qualified to address these concerns than are the staff nurses." If we are to be members of the nursing staff and work together to provide quality patient care, we need to be heard and made a part of the decision-making process. Along these same lines, when we report on a patient's behavioral condition, we are often ignored. Possibly a communication conflict exists. The element of trust is a vital component of the communication process.

We want and need your input to bridge the gap we perceive exists. We want to listen and hear from you, too. Our goal is not to create a rift between us, but to merge and complement each other's skills and abilities to structure a proud and caring nursing staff.

Discussion Questions

1. If you were the nursing director, how would you respond to the counselors' plea and the covert way in which it was formed?
2. How do you think the nurses, administration, and other managers will respond to these allegations of inequality?
3. What actions will you take to meet the requests of your counselors?
4. What implications will this request have on the (1) relationship between nurses and counselors, (2) relationship between staff and management, (3) existing department policies, (4) job descriptions of both nurses and counselors, and (5) hiring practices?

The Independent Contractor

S HADY REST Nursing Center is a 55-bed, for-profit intermediate care facility. Although only three years old, Shady Rest has already developed its own clientele from the wealthy residents in the area and referrals from two neighboring acute care hospitals. The facility has been commended by the local medical society for its superb rehabilitative therapies that include physical, occupational, speech, and recreational.

The rehabilitative services department at Shady Rest is under the general direction of Bob, a registered physical therapist with more than 15 years of experience. Bob is not an employee of Shady Rest; rather he serves as a contractual consultant. Bob is also the sole proprietor of Therapeutic Services, Inc., a contractual firm that provides physical therapy personnel to a variety of home health agencies, the local school system, and local industries, as well as to Shady Rest.

Before the opening of Shady Rest, Bob convinced the owner that contracting with a firm such as Therapeutic Services, Inc., would be more cost effective for the center because of the therapist shortage in the area, the cost of a competitive employee benefit package, and the difficulty of recruiting and retaining qualified personnel. Bob assured the owner that his firm was in the prime position to provide consistent coverage should the originally assigned therapist become ill or be on annual leave. In addition, Bob would oversee his own employees' performance, monitor quality assurance activities, and establish departmental policies and procedures relative to the rehabilitative therapies.

Other rehabilitative therapy personnel at Shady Rest were on independent-contractor status and were notified of requests for service by either nursing personnel or by Bob's personnel. The two groups had a general understanding: whoever initially came across a physician's order in the medical record would take responsibility for notifying the specific discipline by way of a beeper system. Upon contracting the specific discipline, the person who made the contact would document "notified" in the physician's orders section of the chart.

Since the opening of the nursing center, the number of physical therapy referrals had increased such that Bob was providing the center with one full-time registered physical therapist assistant (RPTA), one part-time registered physical therapist (RPT), and one physical therapy aide. Bob was usually available at his off-site office for general over-the-phone consultation with his employees should problems arise. In addition, Bob was on site at Shady Rest on the first working day of every month, when he hand delivered the invoice for services.

Generally, a good rapport exists among Bob, physical therapy personnel at Shady Rest, and the independent contractors providing the other therapies. The independent contractors are each employed on a permanent full-time status at other nonaffiliated agencies and usually provide their services to Shady Rest after hours. Communication between disciplines is therefore limited to specific patient conditions and often occurs in the hallway as the physical therapy personnel are leaving and the other therapists are just beginning their duties.

In March, Bob went out of town for two weeks, but before he left he appointed the RPT to manage the office. Consequently, the RPTA and another aide would be responsible for providing the majority of patient care during Bob's absence and any new referrals would be held for the RPT to cover Saturday. The RPT would also then retroactively cosign the RPTA's notes for the previous week.

During Bob's absence, Shady Rest received a high volume of referrals, which kept the center constantly busy and its staff overworked. The RPT decreased his hours at Shady Rest from five to ten hours a week to two to four hours a week because of office responsibilities, and the RPTA and the aide worked 50 to 60 hours to keep up with the referrals. At the same time, the occupational therapist (OT) was unexpectedly called out of town for five days. The OT notified the owner of the facility, who in turn notified the RPTA of the OT's absence.

While the OT was out of town, an order was placed into the department for a fine-motor-skill evaluation. The prescribing doctor documented the written order in the patient's chart, and the aide, unaware of the OT's absense, relayed the order via beeper to the OT and informed the RPTA of the order. Already overwhelmed by the amount of work she had to do, the RPTA sent for the patient, performed an observatory evaluation of the patient's performance using the Purdue Pegboard Test of Manual Dexterity, and noted her observations into the medical record.

The OT returned to Shady Rest the next day to find the patient's chart and the RPTA's report about the patient's fine-motor status. Realizing that the RPTA was not qualified to perform the test and that such an action was against licensure laws and the professional code of ethics, the OT proceeded to the physical therapy department to inquire but found that the RPTA had not shown up for work. On investigation, the OT further found that the RPTA had been involved in an automobile accident the previous evening and would not be available for questioning for quite some time. The OT must decide what course of action should be taken to prevent this illegal evaluation incident from recurring.

Discussion Questions

1. To whom can the OT turn to help him rectify the matter at hand? Explain your answer.
2. Who is responsible for the mistake and how should this person(s) be handled?
3. Should Bob have informed everyone at Shady Rest of his absence and that the RPT was his temporary replacement? Why?
4. You are hired by Shady Rest as an independent consultant. Your job is to recommend change of processes and plans of action that will help anticipate and ultimately prevent these types of incidents from occurring. What will you recommend?

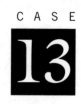

A Change of Leaders

THE HEMATOLOGY department is experiencing low morale, stress, tension, and frustration. Most of the problem is attributed to the department's supervisor, Anne. Anne has not been performing her job well. She has shown favoritism to one employee over others, doesn't work eight-hour days, and generally has an "I don't care" attitude.

The laboratory is facing a major inspection for reaccreditation. In preparation, a mock inspection is conducted by the technical director, and the inspection reveals 30 deficiencies that could prevent reaccreditation. The technical director places Anne on a three-month probation to correct the deficiencies. Anne is also told to work more closely with her assistant supervisor, Jennifer.

After two months, no deficiencies have been corrected. Other employees are threatening to resign. Tension and stress in the department are at an all-time high. These circumstances cause Anne to resign. Jennifer is assigned to serve temporarily as department supervisor pending the hiring of a permanent supervisor.

By inspection time three months later, all deficiencies have been corrected, all employees are working weekends, and employee morale has completely turned around. Everyone is working together as a team.

The technical director has narrowed the search for a new supervisor to three applicants: Jennifer, Grace, and Linda. Her decision will directly affect the morale of the department, as well as its stability and future growth.

Jennifer has four years of experience in the department, is a registered and certified medical technologist, and has the support of the other employees.

Grace is a technologist who is not currently working in the hematology department but has a specialist license in hematology in addition to being a registered and certified technologist. She also has the support of the employees.

Linda is the second-shift supervisor in the department. She has 14 years of general lab experience but is not ASCP registered. Unfortunately, there are a lot of bad feelings between employees and Linda, and the employees have threatened to leave if Linda is hired. Although Linda has had good experience with low turnover on the second shift, the staff on the second shift are not as educated as the first-shift employees, and they are not registered.

Discussion Questions

1. If you were the technical director, how would you structure the selection process?
2. Would you include the staff in your selection process?
3. Who should be hired? Why?
4. Your final decision might not please the staff, and if not, how would you handle the possible uprising?

Ugly Competition

U PSTATE CORRECTIONAL Institute is a medium-to-maximum–security facility that houses 1,200 inmates. Currently, each of the two security levels of the prison has its own medical facility located in different areas of the prison complex. The medical department handles all medical needs for the 1,200 inmates at Upstate in addition to outpatient treatment for 100 inmates at a nearby youth correctional facility. The department is also responsible for off-hours handling of medical emergency services to other medium-security prisons.

Because of the increasing demand for healthcare services, the State Department of Corrections has decided to combine the units and build, on prison grounds, an 18-bed, full-service clinic that will be staffed by three physicians, one nurse supervisor, two head nurses, and 12 staff nurses. Previously, medical staff were divided between two locations fairly isolated from one another, but the nurses rotated from one site to the other as needed.

Top-level administration has suggested that extensive changes be made to provide the needed supervision over increased activities and responsibilities. Definite plans have been made to add eight to ten nurse positions, but uncertainty exists about how quickly these positions can be filled. Upstate Correctional Institute has historically had difficulty recruiting and retaining medical personnel because of poor working conditions and the nature of the work. Among current staff, considerable bickering, game playing, and competition is present as individuals seek to gain advantage in hope of future promotion. Further division has been caused as nurses have chosen sides between two physicians competing for the regional physician director's position.

Strong, assertive leadership is needed for the many changes occurring in the medical department at Upstate Correctional Institute. Chronic short staffing and difficulty hiring and retaining nurses require that care be taken in arranging/rearranging supervision of the combined units. Three nurses have expressed interest in the supervisory positions.

Janet, the nurse supervisor, has been in the position for nine years. She is dependable, flexible, and has good management skills. She is close to completing a B.S. degree in health services administration and has 20 years of management experience. She currently supervises Kim and Barbara.

The maximum-security head nurse, Kim, is relatively new to the position and has held it only one year. She is mature, well-liked, has good management skills, and has just completed a B.S. degree in business administration. She also has about eight years of supervisory experience from another healthcare institution.

Barbara, the medium-security head nurse, has held her position for nine years solely because of her seniority. She is immature, aggressive, and not well-liked, but she is dependable, strong, and willing to learn and listen. She holds a two-year nursing degree.

Discussion Questions

1. You are one of the administrators at Upstate Correctional Institute. How will you intervene to cease the unhealthy competition and improve the climate?
2. How will you recruit for the open positions without overlooking the qualifications of the interested candidates despite their distasteful lobbying?
3. Describe the dysfunctional dynamics in this case and explain how you can resolve them.

Hostile Workplace

AS THE new head nurse, Michelle is just finding out that the nurses, nursing assistants, and secretaries on the unit exercise no form of teamwork and are constantly at odds with one another. Each group complains about the lack of help it receives from the other teams.

For instance, the nursing assistants complain that the nurses assign to them all the difficult patients and then do not help when needed. The nurses, in turn, assert that the nursing assistants are not doing their jobs and accuse the assistants of not answering call lights and not assisting when needed. In addition, the nurses charge that the unit secretaries do not inform them when their patients leave the floor for tests or if their patients need assistance. In response, the secretaries argue that nurses do not help transcribe doctors' orders, schedule tests, or answer phones even when the secretaries are occupied with other things and the nurses have nothing else to do. The nurses admit not helping with the phones because they think the secretaries spend too much time on personal calls and expect the nurses to do all the work when it piles up.

Michelle has observed that the nurses and nursing assistants answer only their own patients' call lights and that all three groups harbor so much ill will that one group does not associate with another even at lunch—if two members of different groups go to lunch at the same time, they do not sit together. In addition, Michelle has learned that physicians dislike sending their patients to the unit because patients have complained that their call lights are not answered and that the staff acts unwilling to help the patients.

Discussion Questions

1. As the head nurse, what should Michelle do to eliminate the infighting and hostility in the workplace, improve staff relations, and provide better quality care?
2. What can her supervisor do to help?

Same Hospital, Different Arrangement

TWO YEARS ago St. Anne's Hospital attempted to increase staff retention and satisfaction by offering the registered nurses (RNs) the option of working ten-hour shifts instead of the usual eight-hour shifts. This change was feasible because of the level of staffing available at the time, but the agreement was not put in writing or in any kind of contract form. Several staff elected to try the ten-hour days; two to four people in each of the three units (units A, B, and C) chose to work the longer shifts.

Last July, the nursing shortage became more pronounced, requests for additional full-time equivalents (FTEs) were denied, and coverage for the units became an issue. The nursing shortage was compounded by the fact that competing hospitals were offering starting salaries about $2.50 above midpoint on the hospital's pay scale. Nevertheless, all except one RN remained, probably at least in part because of promises from the corporate level that salaries would be evaluated and adjusted according to market value. In September, the director for unit A asked that there be an across-the-board decision to discontinue the use of ten-hour shifts. The director of patient services determined that this decision would be made by the unit directors on a unit-by-unit basis, because other units did not see the need to switch to eight-hour days. In October, the unit A director decided that the two remaining staff members on ten-hour days would have to go back to eight-hour days to cover the unit.

The director met with the staff members and explained the situation. They were unhappy about the decision but were told that if staffing permitted, they would be able to work ten-hour days on a PRN basis. The two staff members complained constantly about the fact that they were forced to change and the rest of the units were not. They felt that they were being pulled to cover other units, especially because the other two units did not make the change to eight-hour days and had serious shortages. The staff who had been forced to change rationalized that if all were working eight-hour days, nursing would gain nine shifts per week.

In November, the salary adjustments were made as promised. Some staff got significant raises (largely because their pay had been below the new starting salary), and others got nothing because they were already close to the new midpoint. In March, an executive decision was made by the director of patient services that there would be no more ten-hour shifts except for those who required the ten-hour shifts to be able to pursue their education.

Two of the nurses affected by this decision went to the director of patient services and complained that they were losing money because they would not be working the additional four hours per weekend at the time-and-a-half rate. They threatened to look elsewhere for employment either as a permanent arrangement or as additional time on their weekends off. They were told that they could be guaranteed overtime of at least one day per month to make up for the financial hardship. This agreement was not to be shared with others, but within 24 hours the RNs had shared the arrangement with other ten-hour-shift personnel. When the unit directors were informed of the situation, they expressed concern about the use of the word "guaranteed" and about the effect that the additional hours would have on the unit budget.

Discussion Questions

1. What are the major issues in this situation?
2. What should the unit directors do about the guarantees made by the director of patient services?
3. Are there other solutions to the staff dissatisfaction that should be explored?

17

A Case of Questionable Management

MARGARET ACCEPTED the position as assistant director in the medical records department from Diane, the director. At first, Margaret and Diane, who seemed compatible in their management styles and personal interests, had an enjoyable working relationship.

Margaret was well-liked by the majority of her staff and had previously been the director of the medical records department. As assistant director, Margaret enjoyed the low stress level and the hands-on medical records work. She managed with a democratic style and felt it was important as a leader to set a good example. She was loyal to her company and to her employees.

Soon after Margaret was hired, Diane hired a former employee named Barbara. Barbara and Diane had worked together in another hospital, and Barbara possessed good technical skills, which were badly needed in the department.

It became apparent to her staff that Diane favored her credentialed employees; she brought gifts to them and in general looked more favorably on their work. The noncredentialed employees were referred to as "clerical employees."

Margaret noticed inconsistencies in the way employee situations were relayed by Diane. In sessions with Diane and other employees, as in the case of a reprimand for example, Margaret realized that Diane's recounting of the situation was often untrue or inaccurate. Margaret did not act on her thoughts but began to feel more uncomfortable as time went on.

In the meantime, Barbara began to share stories about Diane and the problems she had had with her employees at the other hospital. Because Diane thought a lot of Barbara, Margaret didn't repeat any of the information she heard.

Margaret and Diane enrolled together in a master's of healthcare administration program. However, in the second semester, Diane began experiencing problems with her coursework and dropped out. At around the same time, serious problems began to develop in the medical record department, and Diane dissolved a position held by an employee who didn't realize her position was being dissolved. This situation resulted in many hard feelings.

Diane blamed Margaret for her problems with the employees. During this same period of time, Diane was experiencing health problems and her husband lost his job.

Although recognizing that her boss was under a lot of stress, Margaret began to feel unjustly treated and continued to perceive unjust treatment of others. Margaret began to seek alternate employment.

Discussion Questions

1. How could this situation have been prevented?
2. Identify the sources of conflict and propose some approaches to resolving the conflict.

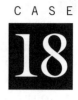

Impossible to Please

JONATHAN IS the manager of an internal department of the hospital. He has no FTE personnel reporting directly to him; instead, as a manager of function, he serves clients within the department. The department has been in existence for one year, during which time the process for work requests has been evolving through trial and error. Jonathan has never received a performance appraisal; however, the administrators and department heads he serves have given him positive feedback about the quality of his work.

Several times in the past months Jonathan has received complaints from internal clients about the level of service provided by Craig, the vice president of the department. As a result of their dissatisfaction with the VP, clients, consultants, and department heads have started to come directly to Jonathan with requests for the specific subservice that Jonathan provides. Craig has been informed, and whenever possible, Jonathan asks the individuals who request service to go directly through the VP.

Craig has accused Jonathan of not being a team player. Jonathan, who wants to be a responsible member of the team, has become increasingly uncomfortable in his relationship with Craig. Recently Jonathan went to an internal resource, Kathy, for help. Although Kathy is officially supposed to be a resource for the nursing staff, she agreed to talk to Jonathan, and Jonathan outlined his attempts to please Craig as follows:

- He asked Craig for coaching. Craig held two coaching sessions and then canceled the rest.

- Jonathan suggested that they participate in the team-building course provided within the hospital system. The written suggestion was never acknowledged.
- Jonathan enrolled in a master's program in healthcare administration (at his own expense) in an attempt to accelerate his learning curve for healthcare.
- Jonathan worked with a private counselor who specializes in business and work-related relationships (again at his own expense).
- Jonathan tried hard—at least from his own perspective—to comply with Craig's requests.

Using transactional analysis, Kathy studied the situation and told Jonathan that Craig's behavior indicated that Craig felt threatened.

Despite Jonathan's continued attempts to perform well, Craig has become increasingly negative. Often Jonathan finds that Craig has put him in a situation where it is impossible for him to please the clients and Craig at the same time. Seeing no other options, Jonathan has finally approached the vice president of human resources to ask for help. The vice president says that the situation sounds like a personality conflict and has offered to mediate between Craig and Jonathan.

When Jonathan arrives for the meeting, he finds that the two vice presidents have already been discussing the situation. Jonathan is told by the VP of human resources that they have decided that Jonathan should leave the hospital by the end of the year and that he should not discuss the situation with anyone.

Discussion Questions

1. Describe the climate of this organization.
2. Can Jonathan be effective or successful in this environment?
3. How can Jonathan maximize his future and that of the organization in this situation?

Combating Complacency

EMERGENCY MEDICAL services (EMS) is an aggressive, county-run system that handles more than 24,000 emergency 911 calls per year. EMS has three shifts, which each work 24 hours on and 48 hours off. Each shift has a captain (supervisor), a lieutenant (assistant supervisor), and a sergeant (scheduling officer). There is also a corporal in charge of each of the nine paramedic ambulances.

Because of the nature of the work performed in EMS, the stress levels are inherently high. Lately the stress has been compounded by low morale and a high turnover rate because of management's unwillingness to change. A noticeable amount of complacency has been observed in the management and field personnel; therefore, improvements in the system have been slow.

One of the staff captains recently resigned for personal reasons. The director chose this time to make widespread changes in the lower-level management. When the new captain was chosen, all of the personnel from captain down to sergeant were rotated to a different shift. The change had been discussed more than a year earlier, so it was not a hasty decision; however, it caused a crisis within the organization. Few people saw it as a needed change and many resisted it in various ways.

Discussion Questions

1. What is your assessment of the director's choice of timing and the manner of the changes?
2. Is there a better solution to the problem of complacency?

The Nursing Shortage

S T. RIGHTEOUS Medical Center is a 250-bed, not-for-profit hospital/trauma center and nursing school in Rightsville, a growing metropolitan area. As Rightsville has grown, so has the hospital, and the rapid growth has resulted in a chronic shortage of nurses. Nurses have historically preferred working at the other two hospitals in town. At St. Righteous, nursing absenteeism and turnover are high, and the hospital has spent a large amount of money to use nurses from a medical personnel pool. The working conditions have become so poor, however, that the nurses from the pool have started refusing to come to St. Righteous.

The director of nursing at the hospital is Betty. Betty has a B.S.N. and has never worked as a staff nurse in a hospital. She has a reputation with the general-duty nurses as being aloof, indifferent, and unresponsive to nursing; she is not liked or respected by the nurses. The assistant director of nursing, Jane, has worked her way up from staff nurse in ICU and is well-liked and respected by the nurses but has been limited in her role by the director.

At the height of the nursing shortage, St. Righteous hired a new administrator, John. John is young with a reputation as a tough, straightforward, results-oriented whiz kid. In March, John decided to address the nursing situation. He scheduled two days of meetings with nurses on all three shifts. Attendance was mandatory, and nurses who were off duty were paid to come. Mr. Olson brought Betty to all the meetings.

During the nursing meetings, John sat next to Betty. At first the nurses were hesitant to talk, but John assured them he wanted to find out what was wrong so he could fix it. He promised the nurses that things were going to change. Betty did not say anything but appeared nervous and fidgeted in her chair. She avoided eye contact with the nurses, while John appeared warm and enthusiastic. Finally the nurses started to voice the feelings, complaints, and concerns listed below:

1. Every nursing unit faces a daily linen shortage; the shortage is especially bad on weekends. There are never enough blankets, washcloths, or towels. Staff go from unit to unit taking needed linens and hiding linens in patients' rooms to have enough for the weekend.

2. Nurses are expected to work three shifts a week and often have to work double shifts (i.e., 3 to 11 p.m. and then 7 a.m. to 3 p.m. the next day). Nurses complain that medicine errors and judgment errors occur because of stress and fatigue.

3. Nurses are expected to care for too many patients every shift. They work overtime without pay because supervisors and managers must approve all overtime beforehand and are usually unavailable or unwilling to sign for the overtime.

4. Nurses are overwhelmed with the care expected of them. They are expected to perform unskilled patient care because there are not enough nursing aides to help answer call lights. Too few unit clerks are scheduled to staff every unit on every shift, so nurses are also expected to do unit-clerk duties as needed.

5. Nursing administration has attempted to use students to fill the shortage. Students provide care, but RNs remain responsible for the charting, and the nurses are concerned about legal liability.

6. Orientation for new staff is inadequate and too short. Staff are expected to pick up a full load immediately if staffing demands require it.

7. The nurses believe their pay and benefits are insufficient; they say there is no time for continuing education and that they have to take their phones off the hook to avoid being called repeatedly on days off. The nursing office is rude when nurses call in sick, and they even call nurses back to make sure they are at home on those sick days.

8. Parking is a problem; there are not enough reserved spaces so nurses have to walk quite a distance to the hospital.

After a loud and heated discussion, John promised that things would improve but that it would take some time. Betty said she would work with everyone to help ease the situation.

Discussion Questions

1. Identify the main problems facing St. Righteous Medical Center.
2. How should John correct the problems?

The Interim Director

S T. ELSEWHERE Hospital is a 600-bed, nonproprietary hospital located in a growing, progressive city. The hospital, which is approximately 20 years old, is planning an expansion program to be carried out over the next five years.

When the position as assistant director of the medical records department became available, the interim director, Pamela, hired Kate, who had five years' experience as assistant director in a 780-bed hospital. During the interview process, there was discussion about moving the new assistant into the director position in approximately six months, and Kate partly based her decision to accept the position on this opportunity.

On accepting the position, Kate was shown where her office would be and was reintroduced to the chief of the medical staff and a few of the department employees. When departing, Kate was told to send her expense vouchers to Pamela so that her expenses could be immediately reimbursed. Kate returned home, mailed the vouchers, and began making plans to resign from her present position and prepare for her new job.

Four weeks after submitting the vouchers, Kate had not been reimbursed. Because she needed the money for her move, she called Pamela, who said the reimbursement should have already been made. Two weeks later, there was still no reimbursement. Kate called Pamela again, but the response was the same. Kate decided to follow up on the reimbursement the following week when she began her new job.

On arriving at St. Elsewhere, Kate found that she had no office and that she was assigned indefinitely to the visitor chair in the director's office. She was instructed to work in all the areas within the department for the next three weeks and to learn each area's functions. The fourth week, Pamela called Kate into her office to discuss her first three weeks, but rather than asking specific work-related questions, Pamela asked about how she was perceived by other employees. She also wanted to discuss personal information that Kate had learned about the employees.

During the next few weeks, Kate observed that only certain employees were allowed to enter Pamela's office. These were the same individuals who ate lunch with Pamela. Kate also observed that when the chief of the medical staff came to see Pamela (usually twice a day for long periods of time), Kate was asked to leave the office. Kate had heard through the grapevine that Pamela was having an affair with the chief of staff. One day, Kate noticed that her travel voucher from weeks ago was still on Pamela's desk.

This situation continued for four months. Kate grew frustrated and bored with the lack of challenges in her new position. Pamela continued to give Kate clerical duties rather than management responsibilities. Finally Kate decided to discuss her feelings about having no office and her lack of management responsibilities with Pamela, but Pamela reassured her that she was doing a good job and that things would be changing within the next two months.

Three months passed with no changes. Frustrated, unhappy, and ready to leave, Kate talked to Pamela once again. At this time, Pamela said that the CEO was not authorizing any management changes and that there was nothing she could do. Pamela said she was sorry and that she would try to change the CEO's mind.

Discussion Questions

1. With whom should Kate discuss her situation?
2. Should Kate resign?
3. How should the problems in the medical records department be resolved?

Unprofessional Administration

ETWELL FAST Company, a private practice that mainly employs physical and occupational therapists, contracts out most of its services to small rural hospitals. Employees are told that the practice is owned by a group of businessmen, but the owners prefer to remain anonymous to the employees.

The president of the company serves as a figurehead, does not participate in day-to-day operations or decisions, but is considered to be someone with whom a hospital administrator can sit down and feel comfortable. Although on a level above the administrator, he is consulted for long-range plans or strategic decisions only after they are made. The administrator, who has no prior healthcare experience, oversees the day-to-day operations of the company and makes all strategic decisions.

Each department is responsible for ensuring quality care, but the manner in which this care is provided is left to the discretion of each department head. Although the departments are given the responsibility to manage themselves, all decisions involving personnel, equipment, patient charges, and other matters must first be approved by administration. Staff are resentful that they are not involved more in company policy making and that all communication is channeled down from management.

Communication from the administrator to the department heads occurs mainly when revenue is down, which results in the perception that administration is concerned solely with money rather than employee welfare.

Several of the hiring practices have caused a great deal of resentment among employees. The administrator has hired several immediate family members for positions for which they are not qualified. These family members are allowed special privileges not granted to other employees, even though other employees recognize that the family members are not doing their jobs properly. In addition, the administration promises promotions to prospective and current employees, knowing that the positions are not available and will not become available. Employees become frustrated and discontented when they do not receive what they are promised.

Turnover and absenteeism have been extremely high. The administrator refuses to admit that there is a problem. She rationalizes the situation by stating that the high turnover rate is a result of the high demand for physical therapists; however, the turnover rate is too high to attribute solely to the job market.

Recently Getwell Fast Company has spent considerable amounts investing in unsuccessful ventures. The company has also recently lost its largest and most productive contract with Quick Rehabilitation Facility. Administration is bitter toward the company that won the contract and takes every opportunity to strike out at them. The administration's manner has been less than professional.

Discussion Questions

1. What are the main problems with Getwell Fast Company?
2. Describe an optimal organizational chart for the company.
3. What steps could be taken to retain personnel?

23

The Overbearing Manager

W E TREAT You Therapy Services is a small, locally owned company that provides physical and occupational therapy services on a contractual basis to area healthcare organizations. It presently provides therapy services to small acute care hospitals, nursing homes, a rehabilitation center, and a center for physically and mentally handicapped adults. The administrator, Suzanne, is 45 years old with a strong background in financial management; however, she has never been involved in any type of healthcare organization. Since her hiring almost two years ago, Suzanne has done her homework and learned a great deal about therapy services and healthcare, and she has brought rapid growth and change to the company. However, Suzanne feels there is one best way to manage—her way. She demands a maximum amount of secrecy and discretion and is less than professional in her people skills.

Rachel is a 27-year-old registered physical therapist. She has been with We Treat You Therapy Services a little more than two years. She was hired by Suzanne's predecessor as a department head for one of the company's hospital physical therapy contracts. She held only staff positions prior to her employment with We Treat You.

Suzanne had been in place as administrator with Therapy Services only six months when she created an upper-level management position for Rachel, reasoning that (1) she wanted to decrease her own workload; (2) she felt Rachel did not perform well as department head; and (3) she liked Rachel and felt she could mold her into an assistant administrator. Rachel was given the title "therapy services coordinator." She had no formal written job description, but she was given responsibility for ordering equipment for all departments, equipment repairs, writing a corporate personnel manual, overseeing quality assurance in each department, and regularly performing clinical services in two nursing homes and any other department as needed.

Prior to promoting Rachel, Suzanne was the troubleshooter for the department heads and other staff. On giving Rachel the above responsibilities, Suzanne informed Rachel that all final decisions must go through her.

Suzanne has continued to have meetings with the department heads and other staff members to discuss things that were now Rachel's responsibility. When Rachel calls a department head concerning a problem or situation, she often finds that Suzanne has already handled the situation without communicating this fact to her. Rachel feels that she will never gain the respect of her former peers if Suzanne continues to override her judgments and decisions and refuses to delegate and communicate.

Rachel has grown extremely frustrated. She does not agree with many of the company's secrets and feels she is being used and ridiculed by management and peers. She finds it difficult to maintain a positive attitude and the necessary image for We Treat You Therapy Services because of her anger and frustration.

Discussion Questions

1. What should Rachel do to improve communication with Suzanne?
2. How can Rachel gain authority and responsibility?
3. Should Rachel voice her complaints? To whom?
4. How could Suzanne improve her management skills?

Promoting Affirmatively

A STATE agency posted the following job announcement:

> Position: Supervisor of Casework Services; Qualifications: Bachelor's degree in one of the social sciences or related field or six years work-related experience in a social service or a combination of education and experience. Position open until filled.

Debbie, Mary, and James were all caseworkers in the department and decided to apply for the position. Debbie had worked for the agency for six years in casework services but did not possess a college degree. Mary, who had a college degree, had been with the agency for a year. James had a college degree, four years of work experience, and had been listed on the state's merit register.

Both Debbie and Mary were called for an interview but were not selected for the job. When they separately inquired about why they were not selected, Debbie was told that the director preferred someone with a degree, and Mary was told that she did not have enough experience. James was not called in for an interview.

A few weeks later, Ralph applied for the job. Ralph was employed in another department, had three years of work experience, and three years of college. After his interview, he was hired as supervisor of casework services. However, the department's performance began declining to the point that clientele complained about poor service. Ralph became frustrated with the problems and cited the lack of cooperation among staff members.

One day in the lunchroom, Debbie, Mary, and James compared stories and discovered that all three had applied for the job of supervisor and had been turned down. James relayed a rumor that the director had returned the state's merit register several times until Ralph's name had appeared on the list. As a result of their discussion, Debbie filed a grievance with the state human affairs commission.

The commission found violations of affirmative action policies and the equal-opportunity section of the Civil Rights Act. As a result of their findings, Debbie was to be promoted to the grade of supervisor, and Mary and James would be given consideration for the next available positions. The personnel director was replaced and the new director was instructed to formulate and implement an affirmative action plan. In addition, the new director was to design a program that prevented additional grievances in the selection process, improved employee relations, and solved the problem in the casework services department.

Discussion Questions

1. How could the job announcement be rewritten?
2. On what basis could you argue that the agency used unfair selection?
3. What would be a good conflict-resolution system for the agency?
4. What future problems might be caused by the existing problems? Who should address them?

The Unexpected Problems

DR. HARTMAN, the only cardiologist in Smallsville, has his office with a staff of three in the cardiology department of the local hospital. He has numerous patients but is not certified to perform commonly recommended cardiac catheterizations; therefore, he must refer his patients to other practices in Capitol, a city 30 miles away. Dr. Hartman refers most patients to a large three-physician practice, Capitol Cardiology; in return, Capital Cardiology takes his calls whenever he is out of town or on a vacation.

Dr. Hartman recently began doing so much work with Capitol Cardiology's physicians that they decided to form a legal merger in which Dr. Hartman would be considered a partner of their group but would continue to operate his office. Because he was the only cardiologist in Smallsville, this arrangement ensured Capitol Cardiology the opportunity to serve almost all the heart patients from that county. The doctors of Capitol Cardiology would also see patients one day per week in Smallsville so that Dr. Hartman could increase his volume of patients.

After several meetings, a quick merger was conducted in which the four doctors became partners. The contract specified only some items. Details such as billing, patient charts, and records would be worked out later. The office staffs would remain the same at both offices, all four physicians would be salaried, and the practice would comprise the large Capitol office and the small hospital-based office in Smallsville.

In the first month, several unanticipated problems presented themselves to the newly merged practice. Because the offices were more than

30 miles apart, planning and organizational meetings were difficult to schedule, but many decisions needed to be made. Changes in letterhead stationery, billing procedures, and patient information were made by Dr. Youngblood, president and founder of Capitol Cardiology, and his staff. Dr. Hartman's staff felt alienated because all these decisions were made without their input.

Also, because of the distance between the offices, the office staffs had not met each other; they spoke only on the phone as needed to answer questions, exchange patient information, and make appointments. Both staffs also had loyalties to the particular doctor who had hired them. When Dr. Hartman called Capitol Cardiology's office manager with instructions, the manager never knew if Drs. Youngblood and Hartman had previously discussed the issue. She was not used to following instructions from someone new whom she had never met. Hartman's nurses had the same problems with Capitol Cardiology's doctors.

Also, the office staffs were not familiar with the preferences of the doctors from the other office. For example, one doctor might routinely check a treadmill patient's blood pressure two minutes into the exercise while another would check after five minutes. This difference caused some confusion, especially when Dr. Youngblood or his two partners worked at Dr. Hartman's office because they never had worked with his staff.

When his first paycheck arrived Dr. Hartman was dissatisfied because of the deductions of money owed to Capitol Cardiology for services performed by their doctors on his patients while he was on vacation. These services had been billed by his office. Dr. Hartman had agreed on the formula to be used to calculate his pay, but he had not anticipated the extent of the services the other doctors had performed. He was accustomed to taking home all the profits from his office rather than being paid a check for the same amount each month.

Discussion Questions

1. What are the most pressing issues of this situation?
2. Who should take charge of the situation in the offices?
3. List some suggestions for improvements that should be made.

It's My Job!

ETTY IS an outpatient clerk in a 150-bed urban hospital. Her duties consist of admitting patients for scheduled outpatient procedures, obtaining the necessary verification of benefits from insurance companies, and working with utilization review personnel to ensure that all the precertification information is received when needed. Various staff members have complained to Jean, Betty's supervisor, about Betty's abrasive attitude and the foul language she occasionally uses. Jean was hired six months ago to replace Kate, who moved to another hospital. Betty has a reputation of being hard to get along with and coworkers avoid contact with her as much as possible.

In June, Betty announced she was three-months pregnant and was expecting her baby in early December. Jean told Betty to review the requirements in the personnel handbook regarding pregnancy leave. A leave-of-absence (LOA) form was to be completed by Betty stating when her baby was expected and the amount of time she was requesting off. The personnel manual also stated that every effort would be made to return an employee on LOA to his or her previous job, but no guarantee could be made that the same job would be available.

In September, Betty began having trouble with her pregnancy. In early October, she was put on bed rest and instructed not to return to work. Betty called Jean to inform her of the doctor's order, and Jean told her to keep in touch. Because Betty was not due to deliver for two more months and was expected to be off work at least six weeks beyond the due date, Jean felt she could not go that long without a person in Betty's position.

In late October, Betty had her baby. When she called Jean to tell her the baby had been born, Jean asked her about returning to work, but Betty could not give a date because the premature baby had some problems. She also told Jean that when she returned, she could only work on the days her husband would be home because she did not want to leave the baby with anyone else until it got stronger.

Jean told Betty that she could not schedule around her husband's hours, but she would see what could be arranged to give her some part-time work. Jean then checked with the personnel director to see what Betty had requested for time off. At that point, she discovered that Betty had never filled out the required LOA form. Because Betty had not done the necessary paperwork and only wanted part-time work when she did return, Jean decided to give Joanne, a temporary employee, Betty's full-time job and put Betty in a part-time position elsewhere in the hospital. This position would eliminate her contact with the public and make her less visible to other employees, thereby relieving some of the problems Betty created.

Betty learned about the position change from a coworker who called to ask about the baby. Betty then called Joanne, cursed at her, and accused her of stealing her job. She called the hospital administrator and requested an appointment to talk to him about the unfair manner in which she had been treated and to request her full-time job back. The administrator called in Jean, the personnel director, and Jean's supervisor. After listening to what had transpired and their comments about Betty's attitude, the administrator asked to see Betty's personnel file. According to the file, Betty had received satisfactory reviews from Kate, the supervisor prior to Jean. She had not yet been reviewed by Jean. She had only one written warning in the file pertaining to a violation of the departmental dress code; she had come to work dressed in a revealing sundress.

Discussion Questions

1. Who is at fault in this situation?
2. What solution can be proposed?
3. What are the responsibilities of the administrator and department director in this situation?
4. What are the ramifications of the Family Medical Leave Act, if any, on this case?

The Evening-Shift Dilemma

MASON HOSPITAL is a small, rural hospital 60 miles from the nearest major city and referral center. The area is depressed, and it is hard to recruit and keep personnel of any kind, especially clinical personnel.

Dr. Heriot, a relatively new physician on the medical staff at Mason Hospital, is rapidly becoming the biggest admitter and moneymaking doctor at the hospital. His performance is excellent, and he is well-liked by his colleagues and his patients. More and more, he has been making his patient rounds during evening hours.

Georgia, a registered nurse (RN), is an evening-shift nursing supervisor. She is an excellent nurse, and she always receives the highest marks on her performance evaluations. Performing primarily in an administrative capacity, she occasionally helps out on the floor when needed. Her subordinates respect her, but she has a reputation for running a tight ship and some of her employees feel that she is hard to approach.

About one month ago, Georgia received an anonymous note stating that he was an employee on her evening shift. The letter reported that Dr. Heriot had appeared to be inebriated that night while making rounds. The writer would not leave his name for fear of repercussions. Georgia checked all of Dr. Heriot's patients' charts for that particular evening but could discern no mistakes.

Several weeks later, two of the female evening nurses quit work without giving any reason. Around that same time, Georgia was working on the floor and overheard two female employees talking about Dr. Heriot. A nurse's aide was telling a housekeeping employee how Dr. Heriot had patted her on the behind more than once while they were alone in the nursing station. She claimed that she now took steps to avoid him because he made her uncomfortable. The housekeeping employee replied that although she had not been approached personally by him, she knew of at least two other nurses who had been harassed. She also stated that she had personally smelled alcohol on his breath a couple of times. She tried to avoid him whenever possible.

Later that same night, Georgia walked into the nurses' station and caught Dr. Heriot deliberately brushing up against a nurse. She promptly documented this incident. The next day, Georgia took her stories to the director of nursing and both of them went directly to the hospital administrator.

Discussion Questions

1. What are the problems from the administration's standpoint? From the nursing standpoint?
2. What are the hospital's legal responsibilities in this case?
3. What should be done about Dr. Heriot's behavior?
4. What do you think the result of this situation will be?

The Abusive Patient

ALLY IS a research specialist in a teaching hospital's alcohol withdrawal clinic. She has been working at the clinic for a year, performs her job well, and has an excellent work history. The clinic is part of a study funded by a pharmaceutical company to conduct research and determine the best drug for alcohol withdrawal.

On Friday afternoon at 3 p.m., Mr. Silver came to the clinic. Intoxicated and seeking admission into the program, he had a blood-alcohol level of .28 milligrams per deciliter. (The legal blood-alcohol level for intoxication is .1.) The common practice for the study is that the research specialist stays with the patient to monitor the vital statistics and blood-alcohol level to determine when the patient is becoming sober and thus is going through withdrawal. The research specialist then administers the unknown drug and the study begins. The human body processes .025 milligrams per deciliter per hour of alcohol, making for long nights alone in the clinic with the patient.

When Sally was notified that the patient had arrived, she went to see him. When asked if she could talk to him about his being a patient in the study, Mr. Silver said, "I'll talk to you anytime, sweet thing." She later went to his room to conduct the prestudy interview, a standard procedure. Sally purposely left the door to the room open because of the remarks he had made earlier and began the interview.

As she explained the procedures of the study, Mr. Silver kept interrupting her to ask personal questions such as "Do you have a boyfriend, honey?" and "Can I be your boyfriend?" Sally ignored these questions and continued the interview. She asked him, "How do you feel in the morning after you have been drinking heavily the night before?"

He replied, "Well, when I wake up after drinking, the first thing I want is sex. I get my girlfriend and do it once, twice, three times, four times—I gotta have it!"

Sally told him, "No, I want to hear how you feel physically when you are going through alcohol withdrawal, Mr. Silver."

He said more loudly, "I'm telling you how I feel—I want sex! Everything else goes away if I have sex."

Sally interrupted him by asking, "Do you have a headache or vomit, feel shaky or nervous?"

Mr. Silver then replied, "No. All I need is my girlfriend and a cup of coffee and I am fine. Are you my girlfriend?"

He began to smile when Sally said, "Mr. Silver, I don't want to hear another word about sex. I am here to help you with your alcohol problem and your withdrawal. Do you understand me? Not another word about sex!"

The interview continued without incident for about ten minutes until Mr. Silver said, "I wish my girlfriend was here. She knows what to do with me. She thinks that I am a sex maniac."

Sally tried to redirect him again saying, "Mr. Silver, what can we offer you here at the clinic?"

He replied, "I need someone to hug me, kiss me, love me—make me feel better," and he stared at Sally.

She asked again, "What do you want to gain from the clinic?"

He said, "I told you; I need hugs, kisses, and love like my girlfriend gives me."

Sally stood up, said, "I'm sorry that is your reason for coming. The staff is here to help you with your alcohol problem," and left the room.

She then went to Dr. Masters, the physician conducting the research, and told her about the interview. She stated that Mr. Silver had made aggressive sexual remarks to her and that she was uncomfortable with Mr. Silver's participation in the study. The physician said she didn't think Mr. Silver was harmful and that Sally should not worry about it.

A few hours later, Dr. Masters called and told Sally that she wanted Mr. Silver in the study. Sally protested that she didn't feel comfortable having him as her patient because that would require her to stay at the clinic alone with him all night; however, Dr. Masters insisted that she take Mr. Silver as a patient. Once again Sally refused, saying that she did not trust Mr. Silver and repeating that he had sexually harassed her. Finally Dr. Masters said "Fine!" and hung up the phone.

The following Monday, Dr. Masters called Sally into her office and told her how upset she was that Sally did not take Mr. Silver as a patient and that Sally did not do what she asked. Dr. Master's said that she had not yet decided what to do but that she needed someone who could do the job, implying Sally's job was in danger.

Discussion Questions

1. If you were the research program director and Dr. Masters approached you with this problem, how would you advise her?
2. Did Sally have a right to refuse to treat Mr. Silver?
3. What other solutions could have been proposed?

The Ostrich Employee

SHELLEY IS the supervisor of a small emergency room (ER) staff and outpatient laboratory. Her staff consists of one part-time and two full-time technicians, and they provide coverage for the operating hours of 7 a.m. to 1:30 p.m. Monday through Friday and 10 a.m. to 10 p.m. Saturday and Sunday. The staff also takes calls for the remaining hours to provide complete 24-hour coverage. Shelley works 8:30 a.m. until 5 p.m. on the weekdays but never works weekends.

When the lab first opened, all techs agreed to rotate shifts. After a couple of months one of the techs, Jack, requested to work the evening shift full time. Shelley thought this would work out well because the other two techs preferred day-shift hours.

Unfortunately, Jack's work performance has become slack. At his three-month probationary review his weak points were discussed, and Jack agreed that he needed to be more careful and put forth a little more effort. He assured Shelley of his enthusiasm for this new job and appeared to be sincere. However, Jack continued to make the same little mistakes over and over again. When confronted with these errors, he excused himself by saying he was too busy to complete all his paperwork. He was also too busy to clean up after himself. Shelley also noticed that he either didn't understand or know proper lab procedures. Jack continued to assure Shelley of his interest in doing a good job and improving his skills.

Shelley began to blame herself for inadequately training Jack and for a possible breakdown in communication between the shifts. Shelley set up communication logs at each workstation and another log for general lab information. Each technician was to check this log on a daily basis and initial it after reading a specific communication. Jack still continued to make little errors; some of the errors became documented technical errors. Once a lab specimen was improperly collected and the patient had to be called back for a second specimen. When asked about the incident, Jack claimed that he had not been in the lab, and a registration clerk had accepted the specimen from the patient. Jack had been out of the lab talking to some of the nurses in the ER. Shelley explained to Jack that the outpatient hours were until 7 p.m. and that he was to be present in the lab unless he was called to the ER to collect a stat. Again Jack apologized for his error.

Other incidents continued to occur; Shelley began to think of Jack as an ostrich who kept his head buried in the sand. However, every now and then, Jack would display some initiative by going out of his way to complete a special test. Shelley felt that Jack lacked motivation and began to slide when bored. It became apparent to Shelley that Jack did not take the incentive to find the answer if he didn't know what to do or if he couldn't remember what was discussed. At another one of Jack's counseling sessions, when asked why he did something improperly, he replied that he was unaware of the proper protocol; however, this time Shelley showed him the explicit procedure written in the lab and initialed by Jack. In one instance, after Shelley had reminded Jack to read and sign the communication log, he read and signed both the communication log and the notebook for employee vacation requests, thus giving his approval for everyone's vacation. At this point Shelley began to question whether Jack really paid attention to what he was reading or whether he was just initialing everything!

Discussion Questions

1. What should be done about Jack's lack of motivation and initiative in his job?
2. Suggest methods by which Jack should be supervised.

Harassment?

AT EAST Lab Supply Company, the technical director was asked to suspend a male employee, Jerry, based on complaints of sexual harassment.

Kim, a delivery driver, had complained that Jerry was harassing her. She said that Jerry had approached her and asked her out on a date. Kim, who was married, declined and firmly told Jerry that she was a happily married woman. Kim said Jerry mumbled something and walked away.

The next day Kim was packing boxes, and Jerry rubbed against her in a suggestive manner. Kim decided to ignore him.

Two days later Jerry grabbed Kim from behind and lifted her off her feet. Kim yelled at Jerry to leave her alone, but Jerry just laughed loudly. At this, Kim became upset, and after Jerry left the room, she complained to the supervisor.

After hearing Kim's story, the supervisor called Jerry into his office and asked him about the situation with Kim. Jerry denied everything and said that Kim was jealous of him because he had received recognition for work well done while Kim had not. Jerry said Kim was trying to get back at him.

The supervisor called Kim back into the office and asked her if there was any other animosity between her and Jerry. Kim stated that the only problem was that Jerry was harassing her.

The supervisor called in several other women drivers and asked them if they had any problems with the male drivers. They all said no immediately with the exception of one woman who hesitated, then said no.

Based on this information, the supervisor met with the technical director and recommended a one-week suspension for Jerry without pay.

Discussion Questions

1. Did sexual harassment actually occur?
2. Did the supervisor handle the situation in the proper manner?
3. Discuss the importance of documentation in this case.
4. As a supervisor how would you have responded?
5. What should Kim do in her situation?

The Suspicious Performance Appraisals

S T. PREJUDICE is a 600-bed tertiary care hospital with a staff of approximately 2,000; it is located in a large southwestern city near five other hospitals, is associated with a medical school, and is a clinical experience site for student nurses and allied health personnel.

In a recent review of the extremely high personnel turnover rate, the director of personnel, Otto, read all exit interviews from the past year to see if a pattern could be identified in the voluntary terminations. Surprisingly, he found dissatisfaction with performance appraisals reported in approximately 60 percent of the terminations. A sample of statements from the documents follows:

- "The performance appraisals must have been written to assess salesmen; the questions would provide little information as to whether I'm performing well in my position."
- "It was a personality-matching game every time I was evaluated. If I thought and acted like my head nurse (and did a little brownnosing), I would get a glowing evaluation."
- "My chief tech would run through the department at 4:45 p.m., grab me and go over my evaluation so she could get it to personnel by the deadline."
- "The head nurse in the surgical ICU fills out evaluations on all unit nurses. I worked 32 hours per week and was pulled out of ICU to work in the recovery unit most of the time, but the charge nurses in recovery never had input on my evaluations."
- "Every supervisor uses and scores the evaluation differently."
- "I thought my performance evaluation scores were good but later found out I was on probation!"

- "Why are they done anyway? We aren't paid any more money for a good one."

Otto was horrified and immediately called in his assistant Marcia to share his discovery. She was less surprised than he had been and stated, "Yeah, complaining about evaluations is getting to be right up there with cafeteria food, pay, and parking, isn't it?"

To determine whether Marcia's flippant assessment had any validity, Otto requested information about voluntary termination reasons from the personnel directors at the other five metropolitan hospitals. The results were as expected: pay, food, and parking were the big three, with no mention of performance appraisal problems at all.

Discussion Questions

1. What action should Otto take?
2. Suggest questions for a new performance appraisal form.

Apathy . . . or Sabotage?

J OHN IS the director of the Dietary Services Department for Mid-
land Hospital, a 300-bed regional medical center. Before John took
this position, he had served in similar positions as head of the
kitchen and director of dietary resources in three smaller institutions
over a five-year period. John grew up in a small, rural coal-mining town,
and when he was 17 years old, he joined the army. He served for 30
years running camp mess halls and base kitchens all over the world.
Continuously frustrated by attempts to advance in the military, he saw
less deserving individuals receive better assignments. He ran his mess hall
in a no-nonsense, no small-talk fashion, and he used the same approach
after retiring from the service.

There had been a high turnover in the dietary department when
John took the position. In fact, one former head had retired and another
had been fired in the previous two years. The administration hoped
that someone with authority and discipline would stabilize this area.
Meanwhile, the employees had developed a tremendous sense of apathy
toward their work. Never the highlight of a hospital stay, the food
quality and service had seriously deteriorated, and poor pay, lack of
incentives, and the hospital's weakening financial position continued to
create discontent even after John arrived. The employees in the kitchen
had hoped that one of their senior individuals would be chosen as
department head, and that created a sense of bitter disappointment with
John's hiring.

John decided that this position was finally his chance to demonstrate
his skills. He put his army experience and methods to use right away by

publishing a set of policies that he believed would get his department going in the right direction.

During the first six months with John as head, many employees called in sick. Trays arrived late to patients. The percent of insured admissions at the institution was not high to begin with, and this food situation created a siphon to the competing hospital as staff physicians began to listen to their patients' preferences.

Finally, the hospital administrator called in a consultant to discover what could be done to improve revenues.

Discussion Questions

1. What questions should the consultant ask?
2. What approaches should be taken to correct the problems?
3. What steps could be taken in the future to prevent such problems?

Broken Promises

THE DEPARTMENT of psychiatry at Wintergreen University Hospital was originally organized and managed under a traditional, centralized hospital organizational structure. It was later shifted to a quasi-decentralized management system in which operating responsibilities and financial accountability were self-contained within the department of psychiatry. Additionally, the department expanded its program by creating the Greenbay Institute of Psychiatry to integrate the new decentralized management system into its triadic purpose of excellence in clinical care, teaching, and expansion through research. During the period of preparation for the move to the institute, management and organization were developed but not fully implemented. After the development of Greenbay Institute of Psychiatry, a new facility was built on the grounds of Wintergreen University Hospital to contain nearly all the operations of the institute and provide inpatient and outpatient care.

Eight months before the move to Greenbay, the newly appointed director of nursing, Aurelia, a DSN, began to hold weekly nursing staff meetings to involve employees in the decision-making process, in anticipation of expanding the role and responsibilities of the nursing staff of Greenbay Institute. She indicated that the nursing staff would be able to plan and implement new programs for patients and would receive recognition for their endeavors, that they would have the opportunity to become more involved with the interdisciplinary team approach in the clinical process, could develop new scheduling methods, and would receive more benefits. As the nursing staff became active in this decision-making process by pooling ideas and suggestions, formulating programs, developing a self-scheduling plan, and creating attractive job-satisfaction alternatives, their enthusiasm, motivation, and productivity increased.

Four months after the move to the new facility, staff morale plummeted. Nursing staff were informed that the patient census would increase and patient activity would be intensified immediately, but no additional staff would be hired. The local newspaper, the *Wintergreen Chronicle*, disclosed that the newly opened Greenbay Institute of Psychiatry posted an operating debt in excess of one million dollars. Management structure evolved into a formalized hierarchy in which the director of nursing was no longer directly involved with the proposed initiatives, and midlevel management now had control over staff needs.

Six months after the move, the nursing staff attrition rate was dramatically high. In fact, the number of FTEs reached a critical low and the institute was dependent on nursing agencies and university students to provide patient care.

Three months following this stressful period, Aurelia made a rare appearance at a staff meeting to welcome new nursing staff to the institute. She described the institute's ongoing process of evaluating unit needs and changes to implement one of the best psychiatric hospitals in the country. She added that those nursing employees who had resigned "were not flexible and didn't want to work hard." The few remaining original nursing staff of Wintergreen University Hospital who were present noted her statement with raised eyebrows.

Discussion Questions

1. What are the major problems in this situation?
2. How could Aurelia have handled the situation differently?
3. What should the nurses do?

How Do You End an Unprofitable Business Relationship?

NORTHBRIDGE REHABILITATION Center opened in December three years ago. The building in which it is housed was purchased from a group of Northbridge businessmen who had hopes of opening the new building as a skilled nursing facility. These businessmen had already hired their clinical managers and contracted a local physician-owned physical therapy group to provide physical therapy services.

When Northbridge bought the building, they extended employment opportunities to the clinical managers and signed an agreement to contract physical therapy services from this physician-owned practice. Northbridge admitted patients immediately. The advantages of retaining the physical therapy contract were obvious:

1. The therapists were already on board.
2. The owner, Dr. Tibia, was a prominent orthopedic surgeon in town. By using his physical therapists, Northbridge was almost guaranteed referrals from him.
3. The physical therapy practice owned equipment, which decreased the amount of capital expenditures required by Northbridge.

Initially, the agreement worked well. Dr. Tibia greatly assisted with filling the rehab beds. He openly supported Northbridge, which helped the facility gain support from other physicians. Within a year, however, the drawbacks of the contract also became evident:

1. Northbridge had no input into the hiring or supervision of the therapists. Although some therapists were excellent, other were less acceptable.
2. There were not enough physical therapists sent to Northbridge, and the company was not aggressive in recruiting additional staff.
3. The physical therapists were the only clinicians not employed by Northbridge. Their loyalty was mixed and therefore broke down the multidisciplinary approach.
4. Good therapists were transferred from Northbridge as Dr. Tibia obtained new contracts. These therapists were not always replaced.
5. Dr. Tibia lost battles with Northbridge about reimbursement, so he began referring much of his outpatient business elsewhere.
6. Northbridge physical therapy profits were not maximized by using a contract service.

After three years of operation, Northbridge had developed a good reputation; the beds were full and business was promising in all areas. Northbridge considered the physical therapy contract issue. Dr. Tibia made it clear that he was not happy about the possibility of ending the contract. Northbridge knew it would not be a friendly termination. Would the advantages of employing their own physical therapists outweigh the disadvantages? The advantages included increased physical therapy profits; complete control of recruitment, hiring, and supervising of physical therapists; increased Northbridge visibility with respect from with the physical therapy professionals in the area; and a strengthened multidisciplinary team approach.

On the other hand, they would lose Dr. Tibia's support and referrals, they ran the risk that Dr. Tibia might develop another form of competition for the clinic, and they would incur the cost of replacing the majority of the physical therapy equipment, which was currently owned by Dr. Tibia's group.

Discussion Questions

1. What are the major issues involved?
2. What would your response be if you were the administrator?
3. What are the probable outcomes of your actions?

Is This a Case of Discrimination?

A MY BEGAN employment at Southwestern Rehabilitation Hospital as the director of physical therapy. She had four years of clinical work experience as a physical therapist prior to accepting this position but had no management experience. She began as a solo physical therapist. After two years, the department grew to ten physical therapists.

In September of her second year, Amy was promoted to the position of assistant administrator at the same hospital. In this position she supervised six clinical department heads. Five were males. Four already had their master's degrees. Amy had begun working on her master's degree in health administration but was still two years away from completing her course work.

While interviewing Amy for the position of assistant administrator, the senior corporate management asked if she would be interested in the vacant administrator position in the same hospital. Amy was flattered but admitted that she felt more comfortable with the assistant administrator position at that time. She noted that she would be staying at her present location for two years to complete her master's degree but would be available for other positions after that time. The senior managers appeared pleased that she was attending graduate school and encouraged her to continue. They were very complimentary when describing her previous accomplishments within the corporation. They also complimented her on her exceptional energy and enthusiasm.

After serving as assistant administrator for more than a year, Amy sent her resume to the vice president of the human resources department at the Southwestern Rehabilitation corporate office. She stated that she was nearing completion of her master's degree and was interested in an administrator's position within the inpatient division of the corporation. She indicated that she was willing to relocate. Amy received no written or verbal response to her letter. After a couple of months, she called but her messages were not answered.

During that same period, Amy verbally expressed her ambitions to Bob, a vice president within the inpatient division of Southwestern Rehabilitation Corporation. Bob had originally hired Amy. He had always taken a special interest in her professional career; he indicated that he was pleased to hear of her ambitions and stated that he would assist her in every way possible.

In a four-month period, Amy received several phone calls from Bob. Each time he called, he indicated that there was nothing appropriate for her within the impatient division but that he would line up an interview for her in the outpatient division. Amy expressed her desire to stay in the inpatient division. He stated that she needed to take a position where she could prove herself first. An inpatient center employs 100 to 200 employees. An outpatient center employs fewer than 20 people.

Amy was surprised that she would not be considered for an inpatient administrator's position, especially because these same people had suggested she consider an inpatient administrator's position less than two years before. The corporation had made many changes during that time; it had doubled in size and had brought in several outsiders. The corporate office had always seemed concerned about their image, but concern had appeared to be even greater in recent months. Amy began to wonder if she was a victim of sexual discrimination. She began doing some additional research.

First, she pulled her own personnel file. There were six written performance appraisals. Four of the appraisals were written while she was director of physical therapy. Two appraisals were written while she was the assistant administrator. They were written by three different administrators. All appraisals gave Amy the highest possible rating: "Outstanding performance that exceeds all elements of the job." Each appraisal encouraged her to continue to pursue additional administrative responsibility. Her various merit raises gave her a salary increase of more than 60 percent in four-and-one-half years.

Second, she asked a human resources manager at the corporate office if there was a corporatewide written affirmative action plan. The manager said no and appeared somewhat uneasy about the subject.

Amy's final step was to examine the gender distribution of the administration of the corporation, which included 11 inpatient facilities and 16 outpatient centers. She discovered that of the administrators of the inpatient facilities, nine were male and two were female. The two female administrators were employed at centers that were merely annexes of nursing homes and had fewer than ten patient beds. These centers were known throughout the corporation as undesirable, while the other nine centers had at least 40 beds and were freestanding facilities. It looked as though it was much more common to place females within the outpatient division; seven male administrators and nine female administrators ran the outpatient clinics.

Amy knew that several of the male administrators in the inpatient facilities were close to her age and had been assistant administrators prior to being chosen for their administrative jobs. The majority did not have clinical undergraduate degrees. Several of the outpatient administrators held clinical undergraduate degrees.

Discussion Questions

1. Is Amy a victim of sexual discrimination?
2. What should Amy do?
3. List some problems evident in this company.

The Problem with the Temporary Pool

ENTRAL HOSPITAL is a 400-bed, long-term care facility owned and operated by the state. In January, during the middle of the fiscal year, the administrator initiated an increase in the minimum staffing requirements in several units. This action was taken as a response to consumer complaints about staffing ratios in these units. While some employees were transferred from one unit to another, no efforts were made to increase the total number of staff to offset this increased requirement.

A pool of temporary workers was used to help alleviate staffing shortages. The administrator hired additional staff to bring the total number up to 25; however, the majority of these workers were filling temporarily vacant positions (vacant because of termination, maternity leave, and leave for extended illnesses). The number of temporary vacancies usually totaled 20 or more at any given time.

Not only did the total number of temporary pool staff hours increase as a result of the new staffing requirements, but the total number of overtime hours began to increase as well. This increase was attributed to the fact that the majority of the temporary employees worked according to the schedule of the position they were filling, not necessarily on the days that they were needed the most.

In April, the administration announced that effective immediately, temporary pool staff would not be used for the remainder of the fiscal year. This action was taken to prevent funding for temporary staff from exceeding the budget. Additionally, overtime would be granted only in extreme emergencies; therefore, units would be required to operate with staffing well below the original minimum requirements.

The leader of the consumer group met with the administrator the day after the announcement was made and threatened to contact the media unless both the temporary pool and the increased staffing allotments were reinstated.

Discussion Questions

1. Will the hospital be able to run effectively without the temporary staff?
2. Was the administrator's decision wise?
3. How should the administrator respond to the consumer group's demand?
4. Suggest a solution for the staffing problems in this facility.

The Revolving Door

SEASIDE HOSPITAL is a highly successful 300-bed for-profit hospital located in a northeastern city of 500,000. The physical therapy (PT) department provides both inpatient and outpatient services. In the past year, the department has expanded its services to include public school contracts, industrial medicine, and diabetic footcare and education. A sports medicine program was also scheduled to be implemented this year; however, the opening has been delayed for two years because of a lack of physician commitment. In addition to these new services, an off-site pain management clinic was initiated that required two part-time positions at a separate facility. This arrangement has caused a full-time staff shortage at the hospital.

Joseph, the recently graduated assistant administrator in charge of PT, has become concerned with the high employee turnover rate in his department over the past year. In one year, the department has faced a nearly complete turnover in staff, including the departure of the assistant director and the clinical education coordinator. Marsha, who has been director of PT for the past six years, views the turnover rate as average for an acute care setting. Marsha is perceived by the staff as a poor leader and has been accused of favoritism toward certain staff members. The staff also thinks Marsha has inadequately conveyed their needs and wants to the assistant administrator.

Joseph has pulled together the following information about the staff members who have left the department since last July:

1. July: Holly, the assistant director with ten years of experience, resigned after three years at Seaside. Holly cited burnout as her

main reason for quitting. She was frustrated with her lack of input into administrative decisions and claimed she was not compensated for the extra work involved in her position.

2. September: Leah, a PT, resigned after two years when she was passed over for promotion to assistant director. She was clinical education coordinator, third in command, and the senior staff therapist.

3. October: Kathryn, a PT assistant, left after two years of employment to attend PT school which did not start until June. She resigned early because of job dissatisfaction.

4. February: Theresa, a PT, reduced her hours to part time after the birth of her child and the delay in opening the sports medicine program. Theresa, a certified athletic trainer with several years of supervisory experience, was told by the director that she would not be program director of sports medicine as originally planned. She is currently looking for a full-time sports medicine position elsewhere.

5. February: Darla, a PT aide, left after one year at Seaside. Recently divorced, she had personal problems that resulted in poor work attendance and poor productivity.

6. May: Martha, a PT aide, resigned after being on sick leave for several months because of a psychiatric illness.

7. June: Bruce, a PT aide, left after nine months of employment. He was working his way through college and resigned after receiving his Air Force commission through ROTC.

8. June: Lynn, a PT, was promoted to co-assistant director after the departure of the assistant director the previous July. She resigned when her husband relocated to attend school.

9. July: Dwayne, a PT aide who had just graduated from college, worked only two weeks before finding a better-paying job.

10. July: Janice, a PT, left after the birth of her first child and moved to Georgia, where her newly graduated husband found employment. She had only worked one year at Seaside.

Discussion Questions

1. What factors contribute to the high turnover rate?
2. What can be done about decreasing the turnover rate?
3. What should the leadership's greatest concerns be?
4. How can the PT department improve its organization?

The Obstinate Senior Technician

THE RADIATION Control (RC) Group at Midwestern Medical School is composed of six senior RC technicians. The amount of time required for a junior RC technician to become a senior technician is two years of actual health physics work experience, and the estimated cost to train an individual to be a senior technician is $100,000. The company is undergoing an organizational analysis, and during this time any vacancies that occur will not be filled for at least six months.

James has been a senior technician for four of his seven years of employment with the company. His experience and quality of work is generally accepted to be above average; however, James is a very opinionated individual and often rubs coworkers the wrong way. In the past four years, he has had two surgical procedures and therefore has taken a large amount of sick leave. Some supervisors believe he used these illnesses to avoid undesirable work assignments.

During a recent refueling outage James was assigned a task in the reactor building that he initially refused to perform. Claiming that the additional task in the reactor building would require him to do two jobs, James instead performed his daily requirements in the counting lab. As a result, he was told to comply or go home. He did not leave and reached a settlement with the on-duty supervisor.

James was generally responsible for the operation of the RC counting lab. His duties included ensuring the operation and reliability of the equipment used in the quantitative analysis of radioactive samples taken by RC technicians for required surveillance activities. He was often unavailable to count samples, so the technicians either counted their own samples or waited a long time for James.

Recently, when James was entering the reactor building to perform a task, he was instructed by a contract security guard to come back and use the card reader correctly before exiting. James stated that he did not appreciate the tone of the guard's instructions and indicated his displeasure by blowing a "raspberry" at the guard, using the card reader, and exiting the area. The guard reported to her supervisor that James did not use the card reader before exiting the reactor building and that he had spit on her after she told him to come back.

The guard's supervisor reported the incident to his manager, who requested that the RC manager look into the matter and appropriately discipline James. The RC manager has asked you, as James' supervisor, to resolve the problem with James.

Discussion Questions

1. How will you handle this situation?
2. What is the expected outcome?

Insubordination

RIGHTSVILLE HOSPITAL is a government-owned hospital with approximately 150 beds. When the director of radiology resigned because of a heart attack, Patricia, the inpatient supervisor, was not promoted to replace him. She filed a grievance and lost.

A new director, Lori, was hired from outside the organization. Patricia then filed suit against the hospital for discrimination. This suit is still pending.

Patricia and Lori had a confrontation early in their relationship regarding reports that were not completed. Patricia became irate with Lori and told her that it was not her fault the reports were not done. Patricia has also undermined the efforts of Lori with the other staff. Despite repeated efforts by Lori to solve the problems and reduce the tension between Patricia and herself, Patricia continued to undermine Lori's authority with the staff. Patricia told the entire staff that Lori was incompetent.

Lori prepared documentation to terminate Patricia on grounds of insubordination. The administration denied the request.

Patricia's performance evaluation was due only a few months after Lori was hired, therefore the clinical administrator performed the evaluation. Lori and the personnel director had the opportunity to review it. Following another meeting with Patricia, Lori filed a second grievance.

Lori, the personnel coordinator, the clinical administrator, and the assistant administrator met to discuss the evaluation. The personnel coordinator, who previously thought the evaluation too high, now suggested changes that improved the appraisal. Three items were changed to demonstrate the spirit of compromise. Lori disagreed with the compromise, but it was issued anyway.

In the meantime, Patricia issued a written memo containing confidential material to her subordinates, but Lori never received the memo. In the memo, Patricia openly discussed and disclosed confidential information. Per hospital policy, discussing confidential information is grounds for immediate dismissal. However, the personnel coordinator only issued a written warning to the employee. Patricia defended herself by saying that she did not know the memo was in violation of company policy.

Discussion Questions

1. Identify the problem(s) with the radiology department.
2. Who's responsible for this situation?
3. What should be done to correct the situation?

The Substandard Employee

SUZY HAD been an employee in the radiation oncology department at College Hospital for two years. She was a graduate of their radiation therapy school and had accepted a job in the department immediately after graduation. At the time of her employment, she was registry eligible. She failed the registry exam twice before passing on the third attempt.

From the beginning Suzy had difficulty dealing with the responsibility of her position. Since College Hospital had a therapy school, the therapists were expected to work with and supervise the students. This role was hard for Suzy. On the one hand, she wanted the students to like her; on the other hand, she enjoyed the power she had over them. This was not the only area in which she had difficulty. She could not stand to be behind in her work; however, she frequently wasted much time and effort running around, achieving nothing. Consequently, she made frequent errors in charting as well as in patient setups. Suzy's attendance was poor. Often she was late for work or failed to come at all. Eventually her coworkers came to expect that Suzy would not show up when scheduled on Mondays and Fridays. They were further annoyed when Suzy took sick time to stay home when her dog had puppies.

The general morale of the department began to decline. The chief technician was aware of the problems with Suzy. However, she did nothing. When the students or staff complained about Suzy's poor setups, the chief technician watched her for a couple of days but took no further action.

Discussion Questions

1. What are the most pressing problems of this case?
2. What can the other employees of the department do about these problems?
3. Whose responsibility is it to oversee the department's work and organization?
4. What should this individual do?

The Consolidation of Laboratories

JOY HOSPITAL decided to separate their lab facilities into two sites: a reference lab and a hospital lab. From the very beginning, resentment formed toward the lab employees who had been chosen to make the move from the hospital to the reference lab. The reference lab employees became alienated from the hospital lab because they were given more freedom and privileges.

During the first nine months after the opening of the reference lab, there was much confusion as to the responsibilities of each lab. Employees were unaware of who was to notify physicians of abnormal values, who was responsible for looking up patient results, and who was to handle specimens received by the hospital lab during the hours the reference lab was closed. Often the hospital lab was phoned by physicians' offices in search of test results that were performed by the reference lab, but the hospital lab had no access to the reference lab's data. No attempts were made to design a plan for a smooth transition, nor was an organizational design developed before the move. The employees' confusion was passed on to the clients.

When the administration announced that the reference lab would close and the hospital laboratory would absorb its staff, negative attitudes developed. Many of the reference lab employees felt let down and arrived at the hospital with a chip on their shoulder, but the hospital employees showed no sympathy. Management failed to reconcile the negative feelings between the two groups but instead showed favoritism toward the reference lab by not requiring them to work weekends or cover holidays. This treatment only added to the differentiation and conflict between the groups.

Discussion Questions

1. Identify the main problems in this laboratory.
2. How should the problems be addressed?

The New Computer System

O UR LADY of Apathy Hospital, a 500-bed teaching hospital in a southern city, is affiliated with a medical university. The radiology department has long experienced problems with scheduling and locating patient studies and procedure reports. Letters of complaint about the lack of organization in the laboratory have been regularly received by both the chairman and administration from irate referring physicians.

When the chairmanship changed hands, the problem was approached with a fresh outlook, and it was decided that a computer system would be purchased to manage all radiology information scheduling, patient tracking, quality assurance data, diagnostic reports, and management and tracking of patient records. The systems available were analyzed and evaluated by the chairman, technical director, and radiologic physicist; eventually, an information system from Digital Equipment Company (DEC) was chosen.

DECrad is primarily a diagnostic radiology–oriented system that can be adapted to ultrasound, nuclear medicine, and magnetic resonance applications without significant software modifications. A link between the hospital information system (anticipated for more than a year) and DECrad should make patient registration, archiving of procedures, and patient billing more efficient activities. The means by which radiology's usual activities are carried out for referring physicians, ward secretaries, PSO registration staff, and other hospitals who refer patients have all been changed. The cost of the system was $800,000 plus approximately $35,000 per year as a salary for the DECrad manager. The system was put online in sections, and the management and administration identified the following problems associated with the change:

1. Patient information was often incorrect.
2. Patient information had often been omitted from the record.
3. Daily processes were unacceptably slow.
4. Requests for additional personnel were considered exorbitant.
5. Attending radiologists were given responsibility for reporting all exams.
6. Undictated exams were listed as outstanding reports and were not billed.
7. Outstanding report lists for each attending physician were submitted daily.

Discussion Questions

1. Why do you suppose these problems have emerged?
2. Could better management have prevented these problems? If so, what should be done?
3. What would you recommend the department director do about the numerous errors reported?
4. Would you recommend continued use of the computer?

43

Problems in the Nursing Department

JERICHO HOSPITAL is a 69-bed community hospital in a small rural town. The nursing department is composed of a director of nursing (DON), an assistant director of nursing, an inservice coordinator, nurses, and nursing aides. The hospital also has about three agency nurses on staff at all times.

For some time, the administrator, the DON's immediate supervisor, has been aware of problems but has not been able to take action because of poor communication and lack of documentation. The DON has been causing many of these problems, and the morale of the staff nurses is very low.

First and foremost, the three management-level nurses in this small hospital are tripping over each other. Specific duties are not clear because there are not enough different duties to go around. Each does what she wants. The staff nurses do not know which set of instructions to follow.

Second, the DON has a few favorite nurses who receive the best job assignments and the best job schedules. Those who are not among the favorites find the DON antagonistic when they ask for time off. Some nurses actually work more weekends per month than others. Some nurses get all of the overtime hours—others need the hours and money but are not given the option.

Third, performance evaluations are done only sporadically and sometimes unfairly. In one case, an RN was asked to sign a blank performance evaluation form to be filled out later by the DON.

Finally, the nurses' morale has been further lowered because nursing department employees get paid far below the state average. The few agency nurses who are always there get paid top dollar.

This situation has gone on for two years. These nurses face a dilemma; despite the poor conditions, they love nursing and do not want to leave the county. The hospital is convenient for them. The administrator cannot afford to let the present situation continue any longer because replacement nurses are difficult to find and agency nurses are too expensive.

Discussion Questions

1. What should the DON do about her department?
2. What should the administrator do?
3. How could the nurses help to improve their working conditions and department?

44

Must I Treat an AIDS Patient?

JOHN HAS been a senior physical therapist at Southern General for six years. One day John bursts into Mary's office asking if he had the right to refuse to treat an AIDS patient. Mary, his immediate supervisor and associate director of the physical therapy department, listens in disbelief as John rants and raves over the likelihood of catching AIDS from the casual contact of instructing a patient to use crutches. This patient is waiting for John to treat him. The AIDS diagnosis is recorded on the patient's medical record.

John's argues that the hospital is not strict enough in enforcing isolation procedures, no written policy exists for dealing with AIDS patients, and medical authorities really do not know all the ways in which AIDS is transmitted. In addition, John claims that homosexuals and IV drug abusers do not care about their own lives, so why should he. Finally, John says he is not willing to take this unreasonable risk even if it means having to leave the medical profession.

Discussion Questions

1. Should John be required to treat the AIDS patient?
2. Should someone else be found to treat this patient?
3. Should the director of physical therapy be summoned to make the decision?
4. What policy changes are needed?

Conflict Between Managers

A CONDITIONING care retirement center (CCRC) generally consists of a combination of independent living units (ILU) and a healthcare unit (HCU), which is a nursing home. A CCRC organization is responsible for services to two distinct populations along this continuum of care. Line authority comes from a centrally located administrator. A housing manager coordinates services and activities in the retirement area and has power comparable to department heads who provide such general services as nursing and dietary for the entire campus.

In St. George's Conditioning Care Retirement Center, the housing manager, Jack, has notified the director of environmental services, Phil, that a particular exhaust vent from a dryer in the housing area needs repair. Phil, as head of maintenance, is aware that the situation was caused by the original contractor's error. He has already fixed the outside exhaust vents and is now waiting until the rain stops to fix this particular vent. Unfortunately, it has rained without stopping for five days.

On the sixth day, Jack brings up the yet unrepaired vent in the weekly staff meeting. Phil agrees to take care of it. He does so that afternoon, and Jack inspects the job to their mutual satisfaction.

During the following week, however, friendly relations between the two department heads deteriorate. The administrator calls them into his office to get things straightened out. Each person presents his side. During the intervening week other staff members embellish the story so that both people are surprised by the words credited to them, words they do not remember saying.

Because the vent has been fixed, the issue now is whether Jack acted unprofessionally by bringing up the problem at a staff meeting. Phil would have preferred to keep the problem between the two department heads; Jack disagrees. Requesting the repair brought delay, but presenting it at the staff meeting—the next logical step—proved itself through immediate action.

After both sides finish, the administrator speaks. He agrees that presenting problems in a staff meeting—problems that could not be handled between two departments—is the correct procedure. Jack has acted professionally. The administrator is pleased that this discussion shows that his staff can openly argue their differences. Everyone agrees to cooperate more in the future. They decide to set a routine for the director of environmental services to give work orders from the housing manager immediate and personal attention to any high-priority jobs. The meeting ends.

Later, Jack tells other staff members that the problem has not been resolved. Phil feels that the incident is behind them, that he can work with anyone, and that it will not happen again. However, he is confused about what happened between him and his former friend.

Discussion Questions

1. Why did fixing the vent fail to fix the relationship?
2. Was the administrator's private meeting with the two department heads the correct intervention?
3. Was the meeting conducted properly?
4. Are there other options that could aid in resolving the situation?

The Delegator

C HARGE NURSE Kelly has never been in charge before. Head nurse Mary, who is new to the hospital, does not know much about Kelly's abilities, but she has appointed Kelly as charge nurse because of a recommendation from her predecessor.

After a short period of time, Mary begins to receive staff complaints that Kelly delegates too much—even jobs Mary has specifically asked Kelly to do. Mary does not know much about management theory concerning delegation, but she suspects that Kelly delegates too much. Mary rationalizes that the staff may be complaining about Kelly's delegating because they are used to Mary doing everything herself and not delegating at all. Neither Mary nor Kelly know much about delegating.

Discussion Questions
1. What are the most pressing problems for the director?
2. What steps could Mary and Kelly take to become better leaders?

When the Appointed Disappoints

WOODY IS the director of the physical therapy department at Northwest Rehabilitation Center. Until last January, Northwest used a contract service to provide its physical therapy. On January 1, Northwest began hiring its own physical therapists (PTs) but struggled to fill the positions.

Tom was one of several PTs who was hired. Tom had about one-and-one-half years of experience in an acute care setting and came to work at Northwest as a staff therapist on the general rehabilitation team. Initially, Woody felt that Tom was an asset to the center.

Because of the shortage of therapists, Woody needed a PT on the outpatient team. The PT chosen to fill this vital position would have a high orthopedic caseload. Woody felt Tom had been doing a good job on the general rehabilitation team, and because Tom also had a special interest in orthopedics, Woody asked Tom to transfer to the outpatient team. Tom agreed to this transfer.

Shortly after Tom became part of the outpatient team, he was observed by several other staff members, including those from other departments, to be sitting around a lot. His attitude toward his patients was rude, and other staff therapists had difficulty even approaching him about the problem. He did not seem able to accept constructive criticism or any advice.

The complaints were first voiced by other general rehabilitation team members and physical therapy aides. Tom was counseled about his disturbing attitude and his excessive use of the aides on his team. For a while, he seemed to improve. Several weeks later, however, complaints began again from a wider variety of sources. Woody decided that since performance evaluations were to be given soon, he would wait and discuss these matters during evaluations rather than counsel Tom again.

Within a week, complaints began, not only from people in the physical therapy department itself, but also from staff members throughout the facility and more alarmingly, from the patients themselves. Complaints included the report of Tom's failing to spend enough time with patients and making aides perform the treatments instead of doing them himself, charging patients for one-hour treatment sessions but only providing one-half-hour treatments, being rude and overbearing to the patients and staff, and possessing a general negative attitude about his work and life in general.

Discussion Questions

1. What are the main problems concerning Tom's performance?
2. How could this problem affect the entire facility?
3. What should Tom's manager or the administration do about the situation?

Simplifying an Organizational Chart

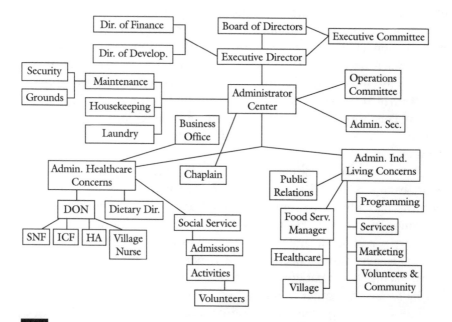

THIS CHART shows the organizational design for a continuing care retirement center (CCRC). Created with input from the board of trustees, the executive director, and administrators, it represents a sincere and wrenching effort to enhance performance and to match the design with the expanding organization's mission and strategies. The design maximizes individual talents and abilities through the positioning of services and linking of responsibilities. The executive director, however, states that the intent of the design has been to protect areas of authority from other powerful individuals and to require coordination among designed services.

A CCRC is a combination of independent living units (ILU) and a healthcare unit (HCU). For client purposes a CCRC supplies retirement housing, ILU, in a community setting linked to guaranteed healthcare in the HCU at a time when mental or physical abilities fail. The benefit to the organization is a dedicated population for the HCU. The HCU presence on campus is vital enough that retirement centers without a nursing care component have difficulties being marketed.

This vertical integration results in a nursing home next to a hotel or, more exactly, apartments. The continuum flows from the ILU to the HCU; both units share common services (i.e., dietary, nursing, environmental, social, marketing) with distinctive orientations determined by unit population. For example, the dietary department, located in the HCU, prepares meals for all CCRC residents. State inspection surveys examine all services rendered in the nursing care facility. They require the dietary department to adhere to any special diets (i.e., low salt, diabetic, low cholesterol), serve warm meals, and provide assistance in eating when necessary. The same food is served to the ILU residents. They eat in a separate dining area with a cafeteria-restaurant atmosphere. The control at the ILU is not state inspection but the satisfaction of the clients. This population decides its own food preferences from what is available, and the dietary department decides whether it is good for them or not.

Another essential difference between the two populations is the living arrangements. ILU residents live in apartments or cottages, pay monthly fees similar to rent, and may leave of their own volition at any time. In contrast, HCU residents are admitted only by order of a physician and are assigned to a licensed or certified bed in a room that is usually double occupancy. Payment may be by government reimbursement. If a patient wants to leave the HCU, an opening must first be found at another facility.

The CCRC represented by the organizational chart consists of a 100-bed HCU established 15 years ago as a nursing home. Within the last five years, sixty ILUs—both rooms and cottages—have been added. Currently, the CCRC is fully occupied and expanding with an additional eighty ILUs, adult day care services, and a health clinic. The number of CCRCs is increasing, and this institution's management is concerned about the low occupancy rates of other facilities even though they do not compete in the same geographic area.

Discussion Questions

1. What are the problems with the design shown in the existing chart?
2. Suggest an organizational design appropriate to this organization. Draw a chart delineating duties and showing the hierarchy of the design.
3. Why will a different model work better?

The First Meeting

ICHAEL, A recent graduate with a master's degree in health services administration, is trained and licensed as a nursing home administrator. He has accepted the position as the administrator of a continuing care retirement center (CCRC). This is his first job in the long-term care field; however, he has 15 years of laboratory experience in hospitals.

A CCRC is a combination of independent living units (ILU) and a healthcare unit (HCU), which is a nursing home. For the client's purposes, a CCRC supplies retirement housing in a community setting linked to accessible healthcare in an HCU at the time when mental or physical abilities falter. The benefit to the organization is a dedicated population for the HCU. The presence of the HCU on campus is vital enough that a retirement center without a nursing care component has difficulty being marketed, which has been true to the experience of this CCRC.

The 100-apartment retirement facility has been open for more than two years and has yet to exceed the present 30 percent occupancy rate. This shortage is attributed to the small size of the apartment compared to the current market apartment size and the absence of an HCU. Construction plans are underway to adapt ten rooms to nursing care beds. This adaptation is to be completed by the end of the year. To resolve the lack of space in residents' rooms, it has been proposed that one unit be expanded into the adjoining room by installing a connecting doorway. A positive consideration is that the smaller units require a lower entrance fee compared to the overall retirement market, and there is an unmet need for lower-priced retirement housing. This CCRC has no local competition. The executive director feels that the completion of the nursing beds and 70 retirement cottages will significantly improve the facility. The center's staff consists of the social worker, the director of food services, the director of environment services, the office manager, and the marketing director. Generally, they like their work and the facility, and they want it to succeed.

One discordant note comes from the marketing director. He is a clock watcher, not a team player. The executive director has questions about a lack of follow-up on leads, a disorganized approach to work, and the recent admittance of a resident with a pet. (The current residents had voted against having pets in the facility.)

It is Michael's first day on the job, and he calls a staff meeting. Michael knows the staff by name and general information from a previous visit two months ago, and he has been introduced to their reputations by the executive director.

Discussion Questions

1. What should be the purpose for a meeting such as this one?
2. How should Michael conduct the meeting and become acquainted with the employees?

The Blood Bank Dilemma

THE COMMUNITY blood bank director, Dr. Strangelove, was following the established protocol when he notified a prominent plastic surgeon that his patient Mrs. Marple—who had predeposited a unit of her own blood—would, in fact, not have the blood available to her in surgery. Upon testing, Mrs. Marple was found to have a positive ELISA test for antibodies to the human immunodeficiency virus (HIV). The usual procedure for a unit of blood with a positive HIV test is that the test should be repeated. If it still tests positive on the ELISA test, a sample from the unit is sent to the state laboratory for a confirmatory Western Blot test. The blood is then discarded, even if the confirmatory test is negative.

Because the unit in this case was an autologous unit, it could be given back to Mrs. Marple; however, it must be labeled as HIV positive and have the donor's name on it. The patient's surgeon, when contacted by Dr. Strangelove, indicated that Mrs. Marple's mental state was unstable and that he did not want her to know that she had tested positive for acquired immune deficiency syndrome (AIDS). It seems that Mrs. Marple, a 65-year-old white female with many medical problems, had undergone multiple transfusions in a larger city hospital during a cornea transplant several years ago.

Dr. Strangelove agreed to cooperate with the surgeon, allowing him to give Mrs. Marple her blood in surgery, if needed, and shield her from knowing that the blood had tested positive for AIDS. Dr. Strangelove called Caroline, the blood bank supervisor at the hospital, and informed her that Mrs. Marple had a unit of autologous blood at the community blood bank, but that preliminary HIV tests had been positive and that the unit could not be sent to Caroline in advance. He asked that she keep this information confidential and that if the surgeon needed the blood, she should arrange to have it sent over right away.

Caroline decided that this could have legal repercussions and that perhaps she should tell her immediate supervisor of these recent revelations. The medical director of her blood bank, Dr. Allen, called the surgeon and informed him that a patient testing positive for HIV could be potentially infectious to the surgery employees and that proper precautions with blood and body fluid should be taken. He suggested that because confidentiality was an issue in this case, the surgery be postponed until the confirmatory Western Blot test results came back from the state lab. The surgeon agreed to cancel the surgery and reschedule at a later date. Caroline was not informed of this decision.

Two weeks later, Mrs. Marple came into the lab for preadmission testing for surgery the next day. When Caroline received routine orders for a Type and Screen test, she recognized the name and asked Dr. Allen how to proceed. He then told her the surgery had previously been postponed, but that the Western Blot results came back negative and surgery was to take place the next day. He stated also that the unit of autologous blood with the questionable screening test could not be sent to Caroline's blood bank and that the surgeon did not anticipate giving a blood transfusion. If a transfusion was needed, the original plan would be followed (that of bringing the blood directly from the community blood bank to the operating room).

Caroline had class that evening and had to leave work, so she left a note to the evening-shift technicians that a Type and Screen was to be performed on Mrs. Marple. The evening shift nurses called the blood bank to say that Mrs. Marple had informed them that she had given her own blood for surgery the next day. The blood bank technicians, following usual procedures, notified the on-call person at the blood bank that Mrs. Marple had an autologous unit and would they please bring it to the hospital to have on hand the next day. The call technician saw the unit of blood in a quarantine status and told the blood bank technicians that she could not release the blood to the hospital.

This situation raised questions in the blood bank technicians' minds, and they began to look for answers. The proper sequence should have been to call Caroline, the blood bank supervisor. If the supervisor could not be reached, they should have called the pathologist on call, Dr. Allen, who was cognizant of the case and a good diplomat as well. The evening shift technicians chose instead to call Dr. Castle, another pathologist on staff at the hospital. She had heard about this case and offhandedly told the blood bank technicians, "Oh yeah, that's the lady with a positive HIV test."

The evening-shift blood bank technicians became enraged. They felt that Caroline was trying to keep vital patient information from them and that lack of such information jeopardized their personal safety. They called the lab manager and threatened to walk out.

Discussion Questions

1. How could this situation be prevented or kept from getting out of hand?
2. What types of policies are important in blood-handling departments?
3. What should Caroline do about the events at hand?

51

Uncooperative Chiefs

HUNT UNIVERSITY is a large healthcare education facility located in the West. It offers programs in medicine, dentistry, pharmacy, nursing, and allied health. A hospital is associated with the school and provides the clinical education needed for the various disciplines. This hospital is a 510-bed facility that serves as the major tertiary care center for the state.

Like most healthcare teaching facilities, Hunt University Hospital has departments that provide photographic services. The Division of Audiovisual Production (DAVP) provides still photographic services as well as art to the university for teaching, clinical, legal, and public relations purposes. The DAVP has two offices. While these two offices are similar in organizational structure and are controlled by the same director of educational services, they are completely different in their production methods and staff attitudes. In fact, there is quite a bit of animosity between the two offices.

One office is located in the Morgan Building, which is off campus and houses the offices of the director of the division and most of the administrative staff, including three secretaries. The Morgan Building site is the center for the production of photographic copy work, materials, and the processing of photography and art. There are five artists and six photographers. One of the six photographers is officially designated "chief of photography."

The other office, located on campus, is associated with the Hunt University Hospital. This office is composed of two photographers who provide on-site photographic services to the hospital and university for whatever service is needed. One of those photographers is also titled "chief of photography." Of the six photographers located at the Morgan office, five are trained and able to go to the hospital site to assist as needed.

Very little cooperation is present between the two offices. For example, problems occur with projects scheduled after office hours. Most of the projects are scheduled with the office on campus. When the two photographers on campus are not able to work the extra hours, the photographic staff at the Morgan Building office is unwilling to provide services. The chief of photography at the on-campus office has been known to refuse a project to avoid having to ask the other office to fill in if neither he nor his associate is available. Even during working hours, the Morgan office is reluctant to provide photographers when the on-campus staff is overloaded with work or when one photographer is out.

Morale among the entire staff is low; unfortunately this problem affects the quality of work produced by the division. Work is often completed late, the quality is unacceptable, and many times the work is lost. As a result, many of the people the division serves have begun producing their own materials. When the division director is approached with these problems, he dismisses them and says that the chiefs of photography can handle the problems. One of the chiefs states that he is simply waiting for retirement.

At one time a consultant was provided to the DAVP by the office of educational services. The consultant worked with the staff for several weeks. When she began to make observations and recommendations to the director of DAVP, she was dismissed and the work was never finished.

Discussion Questions

1. Should the university have two such similar divisions?
2. What do you see as the major problems in the two departments? What should be done to correct them?
3. What can be done to encourage cooperation between the two chiefs of photography?

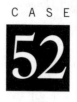

A Good Relationship Turned Sour

MOUNTAINSIDE HOSPITAL is a private, not-for-profit hospital with 200 beds. The medical records department comes under the administration of the vice president of finance, who has risen through the ranks from purchasing manager to second in command. Cheryl, the director of the medical records department, is a registered record administrator with 20 years of management experience in various settings ranging from a small community hospital to a large teaching medical university hospital. The medical records department of Mountainside Hospital consists of approximately ten clerical and technical employees and two licensed record administrators.

In October, Cheryl contracted with Jennifer for consultation services in coding. The arrangement proved satisfactory to both parties, and Jennifer was employed the next March as full-time assistant director of medical records. She was placed in charge of daily personnel operations, while Cheryl focused on physician relationships and problems, departmental planning, quality assurance, and utilization review.

Jennifer passed her probationary period with no significant problems and was accepted as a permanent employee. Cheryl was aware that Jennifer had some weakness in decision making, but felt she was good at handling specific operations issues dealing with rules and regulations.

Both Cheryl and Jennifer entered a master's degree program the next year. Each enrolled in two graduate courses per semester, and each was approved for continuing education tuition reimbursement through the hospital.

Cheryl and Jennifer attended a professional out-of-state conference for several days in the spring. Jennifer exhibited unusual behavior while attending this conference. She appeared to be "spaced out" and behaved inappropriately during meetings and social gatherings. Several comments were made to Cheryl regarding Jennifer's "wild and unprofessional" behavior.

After the conference, Cheryl noted continued behavioral changes in Jennifer. Her job performance declined, she was noted to be sitting and staring into space by various other hospital personnel, she exhibited mood swings, and she was extremely forgetful. Jennifer smiled and giggled almost continuously and responded inappropriately to requests and questions. Her personal appearance changed; she wore the same clothes several days in a row, and her hair was unattractive and unkempt.

Cheryl held a conference with Jennifer regarding the changes in her performance and behavior. Jennifer felt there was no change in either. When asked if she had personal problems that were affecting her job, she stated that her marriage was problem free and that she was happier than ever. During the previous year Jennifer's husband had been unemployed. She lived with her husband and teenage stepdaughter in a mobile home that had been owned by her husband prior to their marriage. She drove an old car with a cracked windshield and rented out her house because she could not afford the mortgage payments.

Cheryl documented this conference in writing and informed Harry, the VP of finance, and the director of personnel that she suspected Jennifer was under the influence of drugs.

The volume of work from Jennifer continued to decline and her behavior continued to be erratic and inappropriate. Again, Cheryl counseled the employee regarding the decline in her performance and recommended she only take one graduate course in the summer semester. When Cheryl signed the tuition reimbursement form, Jennifer listed only one course.

During this time, other changes became noticeable. Jennifer and her husband sold their house and moved into a large two-story brick home with a swimming pool, purchased new furniture, and bought both a new car and truck. She began wearing new large diamond earrings. Her behavior continued to be erratic.

Beginning that summer, the medical records department was required to staff the second shift until 8 p.m. Harry mandated that Jennifer be required to staff this shift. Cheryl communicated this assignment to Jennifer along with the information that she (Cheryl) would be available on the evening Jennifer attended graduate school. Cheryl could not convince Jennifer that this requirement was Harry's decision, not hers. Jennifer went to Harry and complained. She also went to various other hospital personnel such as the director of personnel, the VP of nursing, and the VP of administrative services. She alleged mistreatment by Cheryl. When Harry finally told her it was his decision for her to work second shift, she requested two evenings off because she was taking two courses.

When Cheryl heard what Jennifer said, she obtained the educational request from personnel and discovered that Jennifer had clearly changed the form to reflect approval for two courses rather than one. When confronted with this information, Jennifer stated she understood that she was given the option to decide how many courses to take. Cheryl issued a written reprimand in the presence and with the approval of the director of personnel. Jennifer refused to sign the written reprimand and again went to all of the vice presidents with her story and her recommendation that she should be the director of medical records. She stated it was too late to get all of her tuition back, and she refused to absorb the cost. She then wrote a letter of explanation in which she admitted changing the form after Cheryl had approved the form, but stated that she intended no deception. She demanded that the letter be put in her personnel file.

Twice, Cheryl and the director of personnel approached Harry with a request to terminate Jennifer. Harry denied the requests with no explanation. Harry allowed Jennifer to remain in the two classes and required Cheryl to be on call to cover her absences.

In January, Jennifer accepted a job offer outside Morningside Hospital and submitted a written resignation with notice. After submitting the resignation, she changed her mind and made an appointment to see the president of Morningside Hospital. She told the president that she wanted to rescind her resignation and be reinstated as assistant director of medical records.

Discussion Questions

1. What improper events occurred in this department?
2. Did the director handle them appropriately?
3. What role should Harry, the vice president, play?
4. Should Jennifer be reinstated as assistant director of medical records?
5. What should the president do?

53

Waiting for Retirement

MEMORIAL HOSPITAL is a 160-bed facility located in a small coastal town. The hospital has been privately managed by a corporation for the previous four years during which time the public attitude, employee attitude, and financial condition improved 100 percent. The changes implemented included letting some long-standing employees go and cutting back on the total number of employees, especially in the nonprofit centers except for nursing.

Recently, the pathologist notified the chief executive officer (CEO) of a few problems in the laboratory, problems that chiefly involve the director of laboratory technical services, Faith, and her assistant, Hope. Faith has been looking forward to her retirement in two years, at which time she will be 62 years old. Faith has run the lab without delegating much to Hope, but lately on several occasions she has complained to the pathologist as well as several of the technologists about not having enough time to handle everything. For example, every time lab supplies arrive, Faith opens the boxes and puts the supplies up. When Faith is off, Hope asks a clerk or a venipuncture technician to do the task. Usually she has to face a frown, but the job gets done. The employees are not used to having this type of task delegated to them. Faith has been gone several days lately, complaining of tension headaches and asking to do some of her work at home.

In the meantime, Hope has almost completed her master's degree in health services administration. Some of the suggestions she has offered Faith have been used, but more have not. Faith has even informed Hope that she will not receive a pay increase on completion of her degree.

The pathologist, disagreeing with this decision, has met with the CEO to discuss either switching Hope's and Faith's jobs now instead of waiting for Faith to retire or giving Hope a considerable raise for her good work as the assistant over the last years but at the same time keeping her in her present position. The problem, however, is that Hope earns much less than Faith does, and they both know it.

Not knowing that the pathologist had already spoken to him, Hope made an appointment with the CEO a few days later to discuss her situation in the lab and to ask for an administrative residency. The CEO asked Hope if she would like to switch jobs with Faith before she even told him the reasons for her appointment. Hope stated that she would like to complete an administrative residency after receiving her degree while keeping her present job in the lab. She did not want to switch jobs because Faith would not be able to resist trying to run the lab her way; she felt Faith would treat her with resentment if they changed positions. Furthermore, she said that the difference between the two salaries was not enough for the added responsibilities. Hope told the CEO that there were several other job possibilities at medical facilities in the area, and she was intending to look into them if her job and residency did not work out beneficially at Memorial Hospital. She stated that she would give Memorial Hospital the benefit of the doubt first because they had given her tuition reimbursement even though no stipulation was made for her to remain at the facility after obtaining her degree. The CEO assured Hope that he would think about a solution to the problem and she would be involved in the final decision.

Discussion Questions

1. What are Faith's problems with her job?
2. Should the lab management techniques be changed?
3. What steps should the CEO take in this decision?
4. What career choices seem best for Hope at the present time?

Retaining Technicians

AT CHASE Drug Company, it is well-known that technicians' careers are dead ends. Once hired, they remain in the same job until they leave.

Many of the technicians are very competent. Laboratory technicians require training in the same subjects as chemists and pharmacological scientists, but their training is not as extensive. Although scientists and technicians sometimes work on the same projects, much of the technicians' time is spent performing routine tasks to free scientists for more creative work. Budget constraints keep salaries down, but fringe benefits and pensions are generous.

Despite the generous benefits and great job satisfaction on some projects, one of the major reasons technicians work is to help spouses get through school. Therefore, technicians often leave their positions abruptly. Consequently they leave projects unfinished when their spouses graduate or decide to drop out. Some of the most important job motivational factors—achievement recognition, responsibility, advancement, salary compensation, and career advancement—are absent from the technician's job.

Discussion Questions

1. Can Chase administrators combat the high turnover rate?
2. How can administrators improve the situation with the technicians?
3. Design a career path for technicians that provides incentives for them to remain with the company.

Employee of the Year

J ANE IS a technician in an allied health department in a 125-bed community hospital. She is credentialed in her field and has been employed at the hospital for ten years. She generally performs her assigned work with a notable degree of thoroughness and compassion for her patients and often performs additional duties without being instructed to do so. Jane is well-liked by the medical staff and the hospital staff. In fact, her work and overall attitude have been so exemplary that last year she was recognized as the hospital's employee of the year. This award is based on hospitalwide nominations.

Despite all of Jane's attributes and recognition, her department manager feels that there are some work-related problems. First of all, when Jane is involved in the provision of care to an unusual or interesting patient, she seems to ignore the other, more routine patients. In one recent case, Jane spent an inordinate amount of time involved in an ER case and did not provide treatment to eight other patients for whom she had responsibility. Although she appeared to other nondepartmental staff members to be very helpful in this case, no one was aware that she was not meeting her other job responsibilities.

Jane is also frequently busy with other duties or is up on the floor when less desirable procedures need to be performed. These procedures are, by default, performed by someone else.

Jane's manager has noticed that Jane has a dislike for Susan, one of her fellow departmental employees. Jane frequently criticizes Susan and suggests schedule or workload adjustments that would be detrimental to Susan. Although Susan does have a somewhat abrasive personality, she treats everyone fairly and performs her work in a satisfactory manner.

Finally, Jane's departmental manager suspects that Jane is having a clandestine relationship with one of the staff physicians.

Discussion Questions

1. Are there any significant problems that Jane's department manager should address? If so, what are they?
2. If you were Jane's departmental manager, how would you deal with her?

Who's the Boss?

FRANCINE IS the chief executive officer at Midtown General, a 150-bed hospital that is the sole provider in a Midwestern town of approximately 50,000 people. The director of nursing, Ruby, has been absent from work frequently during Francine's five years at the hospital, and every January, during the busiest time of year, Ruby has managed to be absent for one reason or another. Francine has counseled Ruby many times about her absences and has cautioned her about the consequences of continuing to miss work.

Lisa, the assistant director of nursing, takes over Ruby's responsibilities when she is absent. Lisa is well-respected by the other nurses, is more dedicated than Ruby, and does a very good job when she is in charge. Ruby, however, is well-liked by her staff because of her pleasant personality and is the more outgoing of the two supervisors.

The first week of December, Ruby told Francine that she had been putting off having elective surgery and had scheduled to have it done the first week in January. Francine asked her to wait until March when the census normally declined, but Ruby refused, claiming that her doctor normally vacationed in March.

Midway through January, Francine decided that she could no longer tolerate Ruby's continued absences. A week before Ruby's scheduled return, Francine called Lisa into her office and offered her the director's position. In her conversation, she indicated that if Lisa did not accept the offer, Ruby would still be replaced. She also told Lisa that she would offer Ruby the assistant's position or give her the option of resigning for health reasons. After discussing the situation, both Francine and

Lisa concluded that Ruby would rather quit than step down from the director's position.

However, when Ruby returned, she accepted the demotion. Things appeared to be going well at first, but it slowly became apparent that Ruby was trying to discredit Lisa because she believed Lisa was responsible for her demotion. A split in the staff developed; some supported Lisa, but others who had had a long-term working relationship with Ruby believed that Francine and Lisa had been unfair. The situation began to affect patient care and staff morale, and physicians started to get involved in the dispute. Ruby had gathered support from some powerful people, and firing her might cause some of the most valuable nurses to quit.

Discussion Questions

1. What is your analysis of Francine's decision to replace Ruby?
2. How could this situation have been avoided?
3. How should the current situation be corrected?
4. Should Ruby be fired?

Insult to Injury?

STEPHANIE AND Laura, both nurse's aides, have worked at Mission Memorial Hospital since it opened three years ago. The 88-bed rehabilitation hospital was recently reorganized into specialty units, and Stephanie and Laura were assigned to the neurological unit. Both women work the evening shift, are well-liked by the patients, and are good employees when they are at work.

Four days after the neurological unit opened, Stephanie injured her back and went out on worker's compensation. A review of Stephanie's personnel file revealed that she had been out consistently every few months on worker's compensation. These breaks lasted three to four months at a time. Further research by the worker's compensation department of the hospital revealed that Stephanie had collected compensation at her previous eight jobs, even though she had been well-trained in proper measures to avoid injury on the job.

A review of her good friend Laura's personnel file revealed that she usually injured her back within two weeks of Stephanie's injuries and also went out on worker's compensation.

Although both employees were rarely at work, they had good work records while on the job. According to law, employees cannot be fired while out on worker's compensation, and proving that the women were taking advantage of the system would be difficult. Their managers were unable to gather enough other objective data to fire them. The women are not qualified for any of the less strenuous jobs available at the hospital, and cannot they be trained for any of these jobs.

Mission Memorial is short-staffed and cannot replace these two employees while Stephanie and Laura are still listed in the current personnel files. Their absence requires the use of temporary help that is inconsistent and expensive. While Stephanie and Laura are out on worker's compensation the hospital pays double for the two nurse's aides positions in worker's compensation and temporary salaries.

Discussion Questions

1. What should be done about Stephanie and Laura?
2. How could Mission Memorial protect itself against employees such as these two?
3. What types of policies are important in this situation?

Disciplining the Abusive Charge Nurse

THE BELMONT Psychiatric Sanitarium (BPS) is a 50-bed not-for-profit state institution that receives its admissions primarily from schools, staff physicians, and state agency referrals. Increased competition from private hospitals and pressing financial constraints forced BPS to restructure its overall psychiatric treatment program and synthesize the adolescent and children's units onto one floor. Previously, BPS offered each patient general one-to-one nursing care, and all activities were supervised by the charge nurse, Denise.

BPS hired a new nursing administrator, Karen, to develop and implement a new group-oriented program. Karen, eager to begin the process of designing the program, developed new specialized care and various group treatment plans for individual patient care. Karen also allowed various members of the nursing staff to become part of a patient's team and develop their own care plan for that day. The nursing staff welcomed the changes with minimal enthusiasm and support.

Recently, Karen has overheard many of the workers complaining about confusion with the new system and their frustration with Denise's abusive, underhanded behavior as charge nurse. They complained about her attempts to enforce changes in the overall structure of the unit and about the alterations she makes in patients' treatment plans. None of the complaints were officially stated.

The following week Karen was approached by an aide on the youth unit who stated that he was quitting because he could no longer deal with Denise's behavior. The aide said that Denise criticized his methods of dealing with patients in front of the patients. Karen persuaded him to stay and promised to speak to Denise.

At the conference, Denise was defensive on hearing Karen's accusations. She loudly maintained that she was doing her job as charge nurse and indicated that "someone around here has to know what she is doing!" In response Karen reiterated her verbal reprimand and insisted that Denise improve her behavior.

Later that month, absenteeism and turnover rates in the nursing department became extremely high. When Karen looked into the matter, she noticed that most of the letters of resignation cited Denise's unprofessional behavior and the degree of confusion on the unit as reasons for the resignations. Karen also noticed that the number of sick calls and requests for holiday time were greatest when Denise was scheduled to be charge nurse.

With this new information, Karen immediately gave Denise a written reprimand for her behavior and threatened termination. Denise, shocked by the disciplinary action, refused to sign the written reprimand and stormed off the unit. On that same day, Karen was called into a conference by her supervisor who told her that Denise had made charges of harassment against her. Karen was told to resolve the personality conflict with Denise and do something about the high absentee and turnover rates or she would be replaced.

Discussion Questions

1. What are the major dilemmas in this case?
2. What actions should be taken by Karen?
3. Should Karen have used a different method to implement the changes?

The Flirtatious Physician

SEVERAL MONTHS ago, Joseph was appointed the acting administrator of Medical Central, a rural 135-bed hospital. The chief executive operator had resigned, and as assistant administrator, Joseph was assigned his duties while the selection process was being conducted. Joseph has been at the hospital for less than a year; however, he had been trained in a large, national for-profit healthcare chain and has a master's-level education. Joseph is not a consideration for the permanent position at Medical Central because his previous five years of experience in healthcare do not qualify him for the CEO position.

During this interim time, the hospital admitting operation has been undergoing a "face lift." The business office manager, Nancy, has begun to hire young, attractive clerks with friendly personalities in an attempt to enhance the image of the hospital. The clerks, who are highly visible employees, are responsible for dealing with all patients, family members, and admitting physicians. It was hoped that the presence of efficient, friendly clerks would increase patient/physician tolerance of what was perceived as a lengthy and sometimes intolerable task and that the clerks would improve what was often the first impression of the hospital.

Patty was one of the first clerks hired during this process. She was young, single, attractive, and outgoing, and although she was not experienced in hospital admitting, she soon became a valuable and reliable member of the admitting staff. Patty treated the patients with the utmost courtesy and kindness and also treated the physicians as valuable customers.

Dr. Goodbar is the only proctologist on staff at Medical Central. Highly respected by his colleagues, he is active in the community and as a member of many of the hospital medical staff committees. He is also popular with patients, the board of directors, and the hospital administration. Dr. Goodbar has been one of the highest admitters for the hospital, and he accounts for almost 25 percent of the total annual admittances.

On the other hand, Dr. Goodbar has never gotten along with the admitting office and has often had a gripe with an admitting clerk. However, when Patty was hired, Dr. Goodbar began frequenting the admitting office. At first his presence was not a problem, but soon he became a nuisance to Patty. Patty knew of Dr. Goodbar's reputation in the admitting office, so she tried to humor him as much as possible while not revealing her uneasiness about the situation.

But the situation grew worse. Dr. Goodbar began to ask Patty out, and when Patty turned him down, he eavesdropped on Patty's conversations to find out where she was going after work and showed up there unexpectedly. When Patty checked her employee manual, she found no grievance policy for conflict resolution, only an open-door policy. Patty finally went to Nancy with her problem. Nancy reacted by keeping an eye out for Dr. Goodbar and chasing him off whenever he loitered around too long. This became a tedious task; not only was it unproductive for Nancy to play watchdog, but it disrupted the entire admitting office.

Meanwhile, Dr. Goodbar had been dating the secretary at his private office. When she learned of Dr. Goodbar's interest in Patty, she became vengefully jealous. To discredit Patty, the secretary bypassed her and made referrals directly to the operating room. As a result, patients would show up for surgery, Patty would know nothing about it, and the insurance would not be verified in time. Often the problem would then delay the surgery, thus angering both the patients and Dr. Goodbar, who had no idea what his secretary was doing. The secretary would also provide incorrect information to Patty, which would make Patty look bad. On several occasions, the secretary called and threatened Patty's life.

Patty had a hard time convincing Nancy that this problem was actually going on, and she even threatened to quit. Nancy did not fully believe Patty until she compared the operating room schedule to that of the admitting office and realized that the only discrepancies were with Dr. Goodbar's patients. Nancy knew Patty was a good employee based on her performance before these incidents occurred. She did not want to lose a good employee, but she knew that Dr. Goodbar was an important physician and that his loss would greatly affect the entire hospital. She took the problem to Joseph, the acting administrator.

Title VII of the Civil Rights Act of 1964 states that the hospital is liable for the actions of its employees and that it must provide a nonhostile environment for its employees.

Discussion Questions

1. Is the physician an employee?
2. Should Joseph involve the chief of staff immediately, or should he solve this problem himself?
3. What should be done about the secretary?
4. How should Joseph solve this problem?

The Counterproductive Employee

VICTORIA IS employed as a full-time laboratory technologist at a small rural hospital in a close-knit community. Like many of the hospital employees, Victoria has worked there for many years and in the past had taken on additional public relations (PR) duties for the hospital. This year, however, the hospital has been given new federal aid money, and the hospital administrator, Anita, has decided to hire a public relations director.

Anita gave Victoria the option of taking a part-time PR job and working in the lab part-time or remaining in her full-time lab position. Victoria chose to remain in the lab full-time.

When Jeanette was hired as the new PR director, Anita requested that Victoria be available to orient and update Jeanette about PR matters. However, Victoria failed to be of assistance to Jeanette; not only did she abandon the PR work completely but seemed to be determined to be counterproductive.

Meanwhile, the lab supervisor, Malinda, was not adequately performing her role, so outspoken, overbearing Victoria began to take on some of Malinda's duties. Eventually, Victoria began attending department head meetings as the representative from the lab instead of Malinda. On several occasions when she had a request, Victoria would disregard the chain of command and go straight to the board of trustees.

Discussion Questions

1. What is the main problem with Victoria?

2. How might Victoria have been more involved in the process of selecting a PR director?
3. What are Malinda's weaknesses as a manager?
4. How can Anita correct all the problems?

C A S E

61

A Quality Improvement Program Intervention

VERNON GROVE Community Hospital (VGCH) is a 294-bed not-for-profit hospital in a lower middle-class suburban area 14 miles southwest of an urban center. The hospital's service area is characterized by a gradually deteriorating economy. About 62 percent of VGCH's payor mix is Medicare.

The hospital officials include the chairman of the board of trustees, the chief executive officer (CEO), and the support services department head. The chairman of the board is Elizabeth, a bank president with a master's degree in economics. She has served as chairman for 18 months. The CEO for the past four years, Todd, has proven to be a seasoned, capable administrator and is well-respected throughout the hospital. The support services department head is Joe, who has been employed at VGCH for three years and has served in his present position for a little more than a year. He is an exuberant, aggressive, and results-oriented manager. Joe's department has 204 employees.

The hospital's average occupancy is 67.3 percent, up from 66.9 percent the previous year but down 8 percent from six years ago. VGCH has felt the pinch of prospective payment since its inception six years ago, especially because its competitors have since opened two outpatient clinics and several limited-scope joint ventures.

In January, Todd, Joe, and the chief financial officer, along with the personnel manager, the head of purchasing, the medical records supervisor, and the maintenance manager, attended off-site quality improvement process training at the Quality College. Recognizing that implementing a quality improvement program at all levels of the hospital would give VGCH an edge over the competition, the hospital's administration decided to pursue such a program. Within three months, on-site training for all remaining employees in the support services department was under way.

As early as March, individual quality improvement teams (QITs) were being established and all ten (one for each of the functional areas within the support services department) were in place by mid-April, while on-site training was still ongoing.

In June, Joe was most anxious to speed the quality improvement process. He decided to make a ten-day blitz of his ten functional areas to meet with employees about quality. He was confident that he could motivate his workers, get them to recognize the existing problems in their respective areas, and persuade them to personally identify with the quality improvement process and the new way of thinking at VGCH. Furthermore, Joe was aware of the need to institutionalize any new idea and felt that the time was right because implementation of the process was well under way.

On completion of this ten-day blitz, Joe was satisfied with the progress that had been made in just six short months. Most employees seemed receptive to the idea of improving quality and were quite anxious to begin their on-site training. Several employees specifically voiced an interest in learning more about the quality improvement process, but Joe had noted that many employees did not seem genuine in their personal recognition of the numerous problems he had elaborated in their areas. Joe was pleased that the CEO had made an appearance at eight of the ten meetings to convey top management's commitment to quality improvement.

Joe began looking for some reasonable shortcuts to achieve zero defects a day early. Because only his department (approximately 25 percent of all employees) was involved at this time, Joe felt that it would be sensible to omit the establishment of a steering committee.

Joe decided to let the individual QITs set up their own corrective action teams. He also decided to assist in the quality improvement process by personally determining the major problems and factors to be measured by each QIT and by developing a timetable for each team. This would help to dovetail the activities of individual teams to support an early departmentwide Zero Defects Day.

Joe also recommended to the CEO that the proposed Quality Corner in the hospital newsletter be delayed until the quality improvement process had been implemented throughout the hospital.

By the end of August, just eight months after off-site quality training had started, Joe felt that support services could realistically shoot for an ahead-of-schedule Zero Defects Day. He had not brought this issue up at any of the QIT meetings, but he felt confident that the one-year mark would be achievable. Todd was both surprised and pleased by Joe's recommendation, indicating that while he hadn't heard of any growing pains with the quality improvement process, he was still amazed that it was going that well. Todd approved a Zero Defects Day celebration for mid-January.

By November, Joe started sensing some difficulties in the quality improvement process. Plant operations and the dietary/food service, for example, had moved their measurement charts (showing the price of nonconformance) to less visible areas and failed to put any real pressure on corrective action teams to resolve identified problems. He scheduled the supervisors from these two areas for an upcoming one-day time management seminar. He felt that they would get the message when they received his memo on the seminar.

Joe again blitzed his employees with a round of visits specifically aimed at revitalizing interest in the quality improvement process. To reiterate management's commitment to quality, Todd attended half the meetings with Joe. Employees were significantly more vocal this time around and described several problems:

1. QIT meetings were routinely interrupted and attendance was down.
2. With a few exceptions, the corrective action teams were not used; rather, the QITs engaged in problem solving and affixing blame.
3. Posted improvement charts (measuring the price of nonconformance) resulted in little improvement, with one or two exceptions. In a couple of cases, the charts indicated mildly adverse changes.
4. Only a dozen error-cause removal forms had been submitted departmentwide; seven of those remained unanswered and were long overdue.
5. Only two recognition ceremonies had been held, and those were for suggestion box items (relating the improved efficiency), a program that had existed long before the quality improvement process started.
6. Employees did not have a feeling for what other QITs were doing. Several employees had just assumed that their QITs were the only ones falling behind.
7. A majority of the employees were not sure where the CEO stood on the quality improvement process.
8. Half of the employees expressed doubt that the department could be ready for Zero Defects Day, now less than two months away.

That night Joe and Todd had a lengthy discussion in Todd's office. Joe was asked to make a recommendation by the following week regarding the Zero Defects Day celebration and the future of the quality improvement process at Vernon Grove Community Hospital.

Discussion Questions

1. Where did the improvement process go wrong?
2. What should Joe recommend regarding the future of the quality improvement process?

ABOUT THE AUTHORS

Anne Osborne Kilpatrick, D.P.A.

Dr. Anne Osborne Kilpatrick is professor in the Department of Health Administration and Policy, College of Health Professions, at the Medical University of South Carolina, Charleston, and liaison to the university's human resources management department, working to implement a quality initiative in the division of finance and administration and the university. Dr. Kilpatrick won the 1998 College of Health Professions Award for Excellence in Service; the Medical University's 1997 Earl B. Higgins Diversity Award; and was the first recipient of the college's Scholar of the Year Award. Her research and training has included over 16 years studying and teaching about the management of healthy workplaces and identifying and reducing stress and burnout and eliminating other "toxins" in the workplace. Her most recent publication, also coedited with Dr. James Johnson, is *The Handbook of Health Administration and Policy*, published in 1999 by Marcel Dekker. Her undergraduate, master's, and doctoral degrees were granted from the University of Georgia.

James A. Johnson, Ph.D.

Dr. James A. Johnson is a professor of health administration and policy and associate professor of family medicine at the Medical University of South Carolina. He is also the founding director of the executive doctoral program in health leadership and previously served for six years as chairman of the department of health administration and policy. Dr. Johnson has published numerous articles and seven books in the area of healthcare organization and management. He is currently the editor of the *Journal of Healthcare Management* which is published by Health Administration Press. Dr. Johnson also serves as a consultant to healthcare organizations and networks, where he provides assistance with strategic planning, board development, and organizational improvement. He has lectured throughout the United States as well as at Oxford University in England and the University of Dublin in Ireland. Dr. Johnson earned his Ph.D. from Florida State University where he specialized in organizational behavior and development.